To A gReAt
TRuly loves P
From Ian Samuels

1-8-2023

MW00719351

NURSING HOMES, ASSISTED LIVING

THE GOOD,
THE BAD,
THE MONEY

MY SHOCKING EXPERIENCE
AS A CAREGIVER UP TO COVID-19

IAN SAMUELS

NURSING HOMES, ASSISTED LIVING:

THE GOOD, THE BAD, THE MONEY

MY SHOCKING EXPERIENCE AS A CAREGIVER UP TO COVID-19

Print ISBN: 978-1-66785-662-9

eBook ISBN: 978-1-66785-663-6

CONTENTS

DEDICATED TO
MY UNCLE RUPERT GEORGE B.

I FEEL COMPELLED TO WRITE THIS BOOK BECAUSE after entering this field, I was shocked and horrified with what I have seen and heard. I want people to see what they are committing their mothers and fathers to. They are sending them into a profit-verses-people situation. Many of these facilities are run by companies whose only goal is profit. The managers and some of the staff members are good people at heart and some of that goodness will rub off. But from the top, as far as the owners, it's all about the numbers.

I remember recently, I was asked to come into work on my day off. I told my boss I wanted a bonus for doing that. When a facility is not fully staffed, the residents absolutely suffer. To explain all of this is why I write this book. I want families to understand how these facilities are spending their money. I get to see the journey of people in a way that most people never see. I hear stories from residents about when they were very young. I get to see their final days of life. I get to see the totality of their journey. It gives me a unique perspective.

I also wanted to expose the lifestyles of nursing homes and inform the family members about the financial or psychological abuse they put families through. I wanted to show the readers how a lot of people are being abandoned in assisted living homes. Hopefully, this will ignite some change.

No matter who you are, how tough you are, how rich you are, or how nice you are, you reach the same final destination at the end of your life. I get to work with people who are that stage of their lives. Once they leave my place, they go to their creator or their maker. They don't go back home. And I think that's a very powerful situation I'm in—coming from the inspiration from my grandmother to end up in this field. I get to see human beings at the end of their journeys. You see them one day and they're very nice, pleasant people telling you their stories, and then tomorrow they fall asleep and never wake up.

That is why I said to myself, "If I don't write this book, it would be a waste of a blessing. So this has to be written."

The purpose of this book is to encourage people to think about how you treat your loved ones, and how and where you place them at the end of their lives.

Without being judgmental, I asked myself, *Why would you take your mother and father that loved you so much and put them in a place like this?*

In Jamaica, we don't do that. Jamaica is nowhere as rich as America. There's no comparison. But in Jamaica, your mother or grandmother lives with dignity in their own homes, seeing their family pictures and eating their home-cooked foods. In Jamaica, we have people that are ninety-five or older and still doing farming in their backyards, and cooking. When you go to the countryside, ladies from eighty-five to ninety are still making you breakfast. And then we take turns caring for them in their final days.

One of the reasons I am writing this book is that I want the readers to see themselves in this journey of their family members. Once you do that, you can understand the inevitability of that journey. I think by seeing yourself in someone who is reaching that journey, your reaction will be a little bit more humane and understanding. I just want the readers to put themselves in the shoes of their elderly loved ones as they approach their final destination and see themselves in that same position one day. Maybe we can have better treatment and more love.

I WAS BORN

I WAS BORN AT NO. 3 RAE STREET IN RAE TOWN, A neighborhood in Kingston, Jamaica, that is about a half mile from Kingston Airport. The neighborhood is by the ocean and is known as a place where people come for good music and good fish, enjoying themselves. It was almost like a party town—a place to listen to music and relax. They have different clubs on the beachfront where they would cook fish on the beach. It's a nice area, even though historically, Rae Town does have a history of violence. But over the years, it has gotten better. It's a place where couples come to relax. It's also an area with lots of industries. Investors have turned it into a getaway place where people party by the ocean, enjoying nice music and good food. It's mostly a mature crowd. People from all walks of Jamaica would come there for good music and good food by the ocean.

I remember as a child, at night in my room, I used to hear the vibration of music hitting my window and I really wanted to go there and listen but my parents were very strict, so I could not leave to go where the music was being played. I may have sneaked out one or two times.

Every weekend from Friday until Sunday, I would hear the crowds and the music playing. I would experience the vibration. The amplifiers were very big and very powerful. It was very soothing music which you would like to hear. It was not disturbing to anyone. It's not like people were complaining. I would just lie in bed and enjoy it and fall asleep. I think I may have sneaked out one or two times and gotten in trouble.

These are the fond memories I have of Rae Town. I would see my aunts and uncles getting ready to party all night and into the mornings.

My father was a truck driver at the time for a drinks company. I remember him leaving every morning for work and returning the next day because he had to drive all over. When he was away, I had a little freedom because he was very strict. I could stand by the window and listen to the music play in Rae Town.

Rae Town was just a very good experience for me as a child. It was very sunny all day. The vegetation was very green. People were busy—always out and about and moving around. It was a very vibrant place.

Rae Town was a particularly beautiful, energetic part of Jamaica. The sun would give you energy, and it was just a very happy environment.

If you are travelling to Jamaica, stop by Rae Town and enjoy your first taste of real Jamaican food, drinks, and music. That area is very famous for that. People are close-knit. It's a very nice community.

When I was very young, my family moved to Spanish Town in St. Catherine's Parish.

Spanish Town was also beautiful. It had very green vegetation. It was vibrant. But Spanish Town was more of a suburban environment. It was not a big city like Kingston. It was more of a family-oriented community.

Jamaica is ninety miles from Cuba, and about 600 miles from Florida. It has a population of about 2.9 million. From some of the mountainous parts of Jamaica, you can see Cuba and Haiti and maybe even parts of Florida depending on the location in Jamaica. Jamaica is approximately 146 miles long and fifty-one miles wide, not a very big island compared to Cuba or other places.

Jamaica is a very beautiful place. We have historical customs. There were a lot of influential people born there, including Bob Marley, Gen. Colin Powell, actors, musicians, innovators, doctors. Jamaica is known for its athletes. Usain Bolt, the fastest man on the planet, is from Jamaica. We even had a bobsled team in the Olympics even though there is no snow in Jamaica. John Candy was Canada did a movie about that.

The main industry in Jamaica is tourism, sugarcane, and things like that. Our music is world renowned. Lots of people love Reggae music.

Jamaica has its issues, like any country. There are little gangs here and there just like you have in the United States but for the most part, we are a very stable country. We have two political parties. We used to have political violence back in 1970s and early 1980s, but that's now gone. Rival parties go together and vote together, whereas before, people were being hurt or killed because they voted for the opposite party. Jamaica now is more stable.

Jamaica is a religious country. Every couple of blocks you may see a church, Catholic, Baptist, Pentecostal, Ethiopians, Orthodox, Rastafarian, all types of religions.

It's a secular country where people pretty much get along. It's just the economic issues that we have. As I write this book, one U.S. dollar is 137 Jamaican dollars. The Jamaican dollar is weak compared to other countries.

But we have a beautiful ocean. The Tourists Board is doing a tremendous job in keeping Jamaica one of the top tourism spots.

The Jamaican people have contributed much to the world. I am glad to be part of that history, a part of that people. I am a very proud Jamaican.

Jamaicans who are in the United States are in every sector. There are Jamaican police, doctors, scientists, from every part of the economy. We are very intelligent, smart people.

In relation to the health care—which is why I am writing this book— Jamaicans are in every part of the field. There are nurses, certified nurse assistants, lab technicians, doctors, etc. They are contributing a whole lot to the U.S. people. We are contributing our skills, our strength.

In Jamaica, healthcare is free to all citizens at hospitals and public clinics, which also includes prescriptions. Once you are a Jamaican citizen, you don't have to worry about paying for healthcare. There are three thousand public hospital beds and around 200 private beds on the island. We have 380 public health-care centers, twenty-four public hospitals, ten private hospitals, and 495 pharmacies, which is good for such a small island. We also have a regional teaching institution of the West Indies. Doctors come from the other islands to Jamaica to study. We are very proud of that.

In 2008, the government abolished payment for healthcare. So, when you go to a health-care facility, you don't have to pay anything. You don't have to pay for prescriptions.

But the diet and lifestyle of Jamaica keep people out of the hospital. When I was a boy, many people grew their own food. The farmers would bring in food from the countryside to the markets. These were organic foods with no pesticides. People get sick all over the world. But in Jamaica, we did not have many of the sicknesses and diseases that are in the United States based on our diet and on the amount of sun we received, which is important to human health. And we walk. We would walk to the bus station. We're more physically active in comparison to the West. We walk or we run in the sun and that contributes to our health.

In terms of going to the doctor or the hospital, it's usually minor conditions such as a cold or virus. We're not constantly in the hospital many people are in the United States.

We have a good water system on the island. People are pretty much healthy. There was no comparison between the amount of sickness I saw growing up in Jamaica and the level I have seen in the United States. As a child, I never heard much of diabetes, high blood pressure, high cholesterol. The amount of sickness and disease here in the United States is something I had never heard or seen in Jamaica.

Jamaica is supposed to be a Third World country, but there are healthier people in the Caribbean than there are in the United States, even with lesser medical facilities.

You find more overweight people in the United States than in the Caribbean. I think over a period of time that affects even the genetics of people in the United States. I am not a geneticist. I am speaking as a lay person. But I think people who are obese over a long period of time pass it down to their children. When you go to Jamaica even now, you will not find many overweight or obese people.

Hospitalization and medication, I'm sure, are on the rise in Jamaica, as it becomes more Americanized, with fast-food restaurants, high-carb bleach rice, and non-organic food that people are eating. But for now, the organic way of cultivation still remains rooted in the culture. I am very proud of that.

Right now, we have more than one thousand people over the age of hundred, which is a lot for an island with only 2.7 million people. I think the organic food that people are eating plays a big role in that.

When I was a boy growing up in Jamaica, it was not as if there was food everywhere. I had breakfast, lunch, and dinner. If I wanted anything in between, we would go to a sugarcane field after school and sit there and eat sugarcane and then go to the river to swim. We walked to school; we didn't take the school bus. All of these activities contributed to longevity and health.

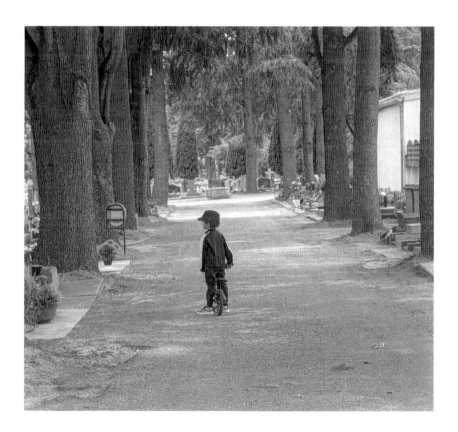

MY MOTHER

MY MOTHER DIED WHEN I WAS FOUR OR FIVE YEARS old. I'm not sure what my mother died of, other than it had something to do with childbirth during delivery of my younger sister.

The only vague memory I have of my mother is her wearing a polka-dotted dress, black and white. I don't even have a picture of her.

When my mother died, there were issues with my father, and he had to leave. It's not my recollection that this is something he did intentionally. There was a dispute between my father and my grandmother and grandfather on my mother's side of the family. It was a big issue over a decision he wanted to make related to me. He wanted to take me but he gave up, or whatever. I was not raised with the kind of care and rearing that you would normally get from your biological mother and father. It was not nice or easy not having that.

Based on the fact that I was raised without my mother, I am a bit surprised that I turned out to be a loving, caring individual. The country, the neighborhood, and the people around me were not consistent in some cases with that. The culture at that time was macho and nonemotional—don't show your emotions. That's the way I was raised, which I was very surprised the way I turned out. I'm not trying to tap myself on the shoulder for being a sweet, nice guy. But to do the job that I do—as a caregiver—you have to be a different type of person. I was not raised that way—with hugs and kisses and people telling you that they love you. I'm not sure if it was genetic, from my father and mother, but I am very happy that I turned out this way. I think the planet raised me, basically, with a little bit of help from my grandmother and grandfather.

Right now, I am feeling very comfortable about who I am. My life is good. I have no regrets or remorse. Of course, every child wishes they had a mother and father in their lives. But I don't think about that. I just move on.

My grandmother raised me. We moved from Rae Town to the part of Kingston known as Spanish Town. It was a new housing development. My grandmother worked at the Spanish Town General Hospital as a nurse. My grandfather worked at Innswood Sugarcane Factory. My grandfather and my grandmother earned enough money to take care of us and my aunt and uncles. Watching my grandmother get up and go to work in a hospital every day was something that I was exposed to as a child and would be a strong influence and example throughout my life.

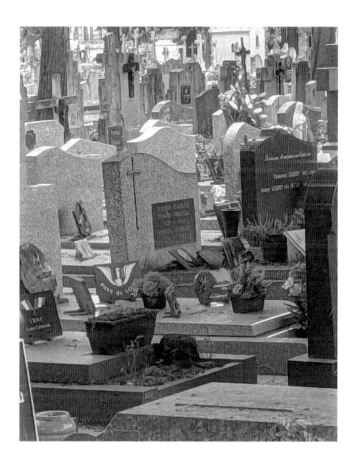

LEARNING CHORES

I HAD A FAIRLY GOOD CHILDHOOD. I REMEMBER THERE
was a train track that went by the river. We could get on top of the train and
as it passed the river, we would jump off it into the river.

There was a sugar cane field next to the river. We would sit in the cane
field and eat sugarcane for hours.

We wore uniforms in schools and I washed my own uniform when I
was young. I also pressed it.

I had other chores as well. There were sections of the house that I
cleaned. We used three different processes. We would sweep every day but
major deep cleaning was done every Saturday in preparation for Sunday,
which was the day when we cooked the biggest meal of the week. For Saturday
cleanings, we would sweep first and then use a cloth to wash the floor with
a bucket of water, and then we would use a polish. It was like a red wax-type
of polish. We would polish the floor, let it dry, and then we'd use a coconut
bowl. It was dried coconut that we turned into a brush. We would scrub the
floor thoroughly on our hands and knees. This was around 1979, early 1980s,
when I was a little child.

My chores included cleaning the kitchen and the porch, which we called
the veranda in Jamaica. The type of lifestyle that we had was very dedicated
to taking care of yourself, being responsible.

It prepared me for a career later in nursing homes.

After going to primary school, I went to a school called Tivoli Gardens
High School.

Tivoli Gardens was one of the toughest neighborhoods in Jamaica. But we, as kids, were safe. Nobody really messes with you as a kid.

Overall, I had a good childhood. There were ups and downs economically. I didn't grow up in a very emotional family. Jamaicans are not very emotional. The don't hug and kiss children a lot. They prove love instead of saying it. They will do anything in the world for you but you are not going to be getting a lot of hugs and kisses. That's just part of the culture, basically. That's why I don't get emotional about things.

In school, I was very average, not at the top of the class, but always in the middle. I was the teacher's pet at one point. I was in track and field. I had a lot of girlfriends. I was in the top tier of guys who got most of the attention. I did get myself in trouble sometimes.

In high school, my grades started to improve. After I graduated from high school, I did little odd jobs initially.

My grandmother was the first in our family to migrate to the United States with my grandfather. The rest of the family stayed back in Jamaica and continued their lives. After being in the U.S. for a while, my grandparents filed a petition for me to go there as well. It was about four years after I graduated from high school.

At one point, I wanted to be a police officer. I went to a place in Kingston where they gave the police exam. I took the exam and passed, but my grandmother said, "No, you are coming to the U.S." So, I migrated to the U.S. and did not pursue being a police officer after that.

I followed a long line of relatives who had migrated to the U.S., starting in the 1970s, starting with an aunt. She made a lot of money and built churches in Lower Manhattan with her own money. She started a chain migration for my family in the 1970s and 1980s. We helped each other to move to the U.S. Now almost all of us are here. I was actually one of the last to arrive. I was not in a rush. But I too ended up coming here.

A NEW COUNTRY

IT WAS A VERY GREAT EXPERIENCE FOR ME TO SEE A new country.

It was a positive shock and awe when I arrived in the U.S. at JFK Airport. I was confused about a lot of stuff. There were roads on top of roads, tunnels, and lights. You could tell the economy was 100 percent different than Jamaica's. You would tell that there was a lot going on here. People were moving fast. There were pretty cars and lights, and you could tell there was growth here. It was just a different world and a bit of a shock to my brain to see all of what was going on here.

Everything was totally different from what I was used to in the Caribbean. The smells, even the economy itself. It took a while to get used to the food. Pizza looked disgusting to me. I vowed I would never eat it. Now I am a big fan of pizza.

When you looked around, you could see that it's a robust economy. Immediately, even before you start living in the country, you get a sense of growth and development. You get a sense that you can achieve whatever you want to achieve. You can do whatever you choose to do with your life. You go through different stages psychology as to what you want to do, what you want to achieve, what you like, and what you don't like. It's a process.

At first, I was trying to get used to the country, doing little odd jobs here and there, and still trying to find my direction on what I wanted to do and where I wanted to go in life.

It was very good, especially because you are new and people treated you nicely the first time they see you. Everybody was polite. Everybody was happy to see you. That first experience was exhilarating. It was very good.

But I went through different stages. I missed the food back home. I missed the culture. Now I was in a new world.

In particular, I missed my national dish called ackee and salted fish. It was a codfish with salt in it. We would boil it and serve it with green bananas and dumplings. The dumplings were made with cornmeal and we would make it into something like pizza dough, but very small and round, almost bite-sized. We would have that with tomatoes, onions, lime, and all different herbs and spices in it and cook it down. We had a yellow yam. That is our national dish.

In the United States, you can find ackee and salted fish in some Korean stores, but it's not the same because they have it in a can and it's not the same quality. It tastes different. It doesn't have that authentic taste.

I missed the food and I missed the environment. I missed the breeze because it was snowing when I came here and there was ice everywhere. I didn't have winter clothing at that time. At the same time, there were so many fun things to do. Food was everywhere. There were so many fancy stores where you could buy nice, fancy clothes.

You would see nice clothes, nice sneakers, and that would add to your joy. I was happy with this new place, new clothes, and even the smell. There is a natural smell that the U.S. has that's different from Jamaica. When you leave the plane and you get out in the country, you notice it. It's not bad or dirty, just different.

I was open-minded about the United States. I took my time to analyze things before I jumped to conclusions. As I moved around in the U.S and experienced new things and tried different things, I started to understand the psychology of people and the system here as it relates to human functionality, psychology, the economy, and the do's and don'ts of life, which is the most important part. The United States is a free country, but it is a country with laws and you have to stay in your lane and obey those laws.

You can take out a loan, but you have to pay it back.

I was trying different things, but I was not necessarily happy with New York. I was in the Bronx and there was a lot of poverty. I saw old cars on the road. I saw gangs and guns.

LEAVING NEW YORK

I JUST DID NOT LIKE LIVING IN NEW YORK, PARTICU-
larly the Bronx. People there were more hardened. One day, I just packed my stuff and left. I didn't know where I was going. I just left.

I had a friend in New Brunswick, New Jersey, and I said to him, "Look, man, I need to get out of here. I can't live around all this stuff. Guys on the corner selling weed and old cars and people hanging out on the street."

It reminded me of the bad parts of Jamaica. I'm supposed to be in America. I didn't want to deal with it. I didn't want to be caught up in it. I didn't want to be a product of that environment.

So, I packed my bags and headed to New Jersey. I wasn't sure how I was going to live or where I was going to work, but I had to go. In Central and South Jersey, there isn't as much public transportation as there is in New York. You have to get a car. You have no choice but to get your life together.

It was destiny. If I had stayed in New York, I would not have been in the medical field, that's for sure. By moving to New Jersey, not only did I get a better life, but I got a more stable life where I would always be guaranteed a job. One morning when I first arrived in New Jersey, I was walking, and I saw all these people in front of a big building. It was a school, and they were wearing white uniforms and I asked myself, "What do they do?" Every morning I kept seeing them.

They looked professional, and it turned out to be a school that trained people to be nursing assistants. You learned anatomy, physiology, urology. You could use this type of knowledge to work in a hospital.

I went in and investigated, and I signed up the same day because it was a cool career. I was thinking about the future and I knew that this was a job and a skill that would always be in demand anywhere.

And so, I went to the school for three months. It was called Suburban Technical School for Nursing. I took the course, did well, and graduated. My instructor really liked me and I graduated with good scores and started working in health care.

At first, it was not easy to get a job without experience but there are places that would hire you.

Right after graduation, I had to take the state board exams to get my license. Then I took my certification exam after that.

I was already inspired by the health-care occupation from seeing my grandmother work in a hospital. I was very young, but I remember hearing her talk about caring for patients. Some of the small procedures may be different in Jamaica, but as far as the concept of the industry, I understood that from my grandmother. But I was the first in my family to work in the medical field in the United States. Even to this day, I am the only one. I had to learn a lot and adapt to a new culture. The first couple of years was not easy.

GETTING A JOB
RIGHT OFF THE BAT

AFTER I GOT MY CERTIFICATION, I WAS HIRED AT A nursing home as a certified nursing assistant (CNA). There was a big demand at that time for people in the health-care field, especially males because of their physical strength. Your first job is not necessarily a high-paying position, but the pay goes up as you gain experience.

At first, you follow an experienced employee, and you watch what they do, because every facility has its own procedures and ways of doing things.

The first day was orientation. You do a lot of paperwork, and watch a lot of videos about the Residents Bill of Rights, infection control, and company policy. You learn about how to prevent back injuries, how to lift things properly. Then they give you a tour of the building and introduce you to the staff. The heads of all departments would come and introduce themselves and give you a pep talk on how they started out in housekeeping and now they were the director. Then you go back for more paperwork.

You are assigned a preceptor to shadow who will show you the ropes.

That's when reality kicked in. My preceptor was taking care of twelve to thirteen people. These human beings all had their own needs, wants, likes, and diagnoses. They had different health issues such as Alzheimer's, dementia, and psychoses, and all were taking different drugs. There were so many different situations. My preceptor had to help all these patients, and they would ring the bell at different times for assistance.

I was shocked by the reality of the situation. I had never seen people in such a state. Even though the U.S. was a modern, wealthy country, it was surprising to see, for the first time, people who were so vulnerable and needed so much help. And it was surprising to see there were not enough supplies or personnel to help them.

Even when you need to take a break, it's not easy to take one, especially in the morning. If you do take a break, you're going to fall behind. Now we do digital documentation of patient care. Back then, we were doing documentation on paper. That took a long time.

There was no time to do the documentation correctly. If there was a change in the patient's status, behavior, or functionality that particular day, you didn't have time for that. In order to get done for the day, you basically must copy what the previous CNA wrote. The legal document you are filling out is a lie. You basically lie every day on the paperwork. You can't go by the book; you can't tell the truth; you just have to do what you need to do. This is the inside reality.

My preceptor did her best. There were other staff, but each person had their own work to do, so they couldn't always stop and answer your call if you were suddenly overloaded with requests. For example, you would be helping a patient in Room 220A but the patient in room 221B is ringing the bell for help.

I was starting to see for myself now that it was not going to be easy. I was working different shifts, usually seven a.m. to three p.m. or three p.m. to eleven. Occasionally, I did have to work midnight to seven in the morning, but it wasn't something I liked.

MY CAREER PROGRESSION

A LOT OF CNAS DO NOT LIKE TO TRAIN YOU. THEY SEE that you're new and think you're holding them back. They want to get the day over with. They're tired. They feel like they have to go by the book during training.

In this field, nobody wants to go by the book. One of the reasons is, you can't get your work done if you go by the book. When you have twelve, thirteen, fourteen people you are assigned to help, who has time to go by the book? Every room you entered, if you looked at the amount of work that needed to be done and compared that to the reality of the situation, you realize that it can't be done. You would be with one patient and another patient presses the call light for assistance and there may not be another person to answer that.

If you go by what the health department expects of you, you can never get all your work done in time. You have company pressure to get the job done in a certain time, and if you don't get your job done, then there's a snowball of issues that come up.

So, I was shadowing with the preceptor, and you can tell the person— even though they were trying to be nice—really didn't want to do this. They are having to take shortcuts to survive and they aren't sure if they can trust you.

While they are training you, the preceptors must do things like knock on patients' doors, wash their hands, put on gloves—stuff that nobody has time for in the real world as far as nursing homes or geriatrics, extended-care facilities are concerned.

I'm with the preceptor and they hit us with an assignment sheet. There are patients who can't walk, others who can't talk. There are patients with tracheotomies, colostomies. You are going through all the thirteen different people and trying to decide which patients will take priority.

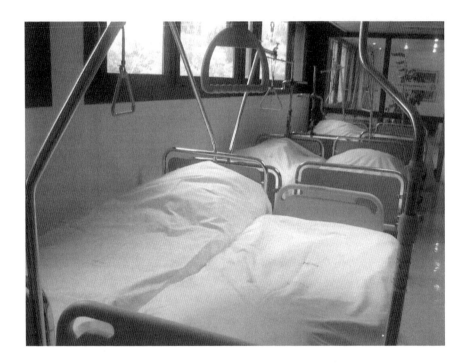

SETTING PRIORITIES

YOU HAVE TO PRIORITIZE, BUT IT'S 100 PERCENT unpredictable. While a patient may be in a good mood today, tomorrow might be a disaster. There could be side effects from medications, or they could be upset about something.

Meanwhile, you have someone who needs to be turned so they won't get bed sores. You may have to turn them every two hours or so. You have a lot going on at once. I'm with the preceptor and I see her running back and forth. You are supposed to take two fifteen-minute breaks and another break for lunch. In reality, I could see those breaks were not going to happen. There was just too much work to do.

In fact, you can't even think about taking a break. You run back and forth, trying to get people breakfast. Then you must get them dressed. You may have two or three showers to give. If the patient can't stand, you must use the lift machine to put them on a chair, roll them into the shower, and that shower is going to take a decent thirty to thirty-five minutes if you're fast. If you're slow, I would say at least forty-five minutes for a good shower. You have to call for help to use the lift machine because you're not allowed to use the machine on your own.

The CNA is under a lot of pressure, physically and mentally.

You get people up for breakfast and then take them out to the dining room. Then you have a list of people who aren't able to go to the dining room that you have to feed. You have to sit with them and feed them. Some struggle to eat. They just don't have any appetite. They're losing weight and they get dehydrated, and it snowballs; their health deteriorates. For me, that first day was nerve-wracking because now I'm seeing the reality of time. These are humans, and you start to feel very bad for them. But then you're pressured because you only have so much time.

I didn't have experience, but I learned fast. My orientation only lasted for five days. My prefector told my supervisor, "This guy's good. He is fast and strong."

I received my first assignment—thirteen residents of my own. Males get the hardest patients. There is a lot of sexism in the CNA industry because men are strong, and they can lift. It was a Friday when I got my own patient assignments. I had people to shower and feed. Now I was on my own. That first day was no joke. I was running back and forth, all the time watching the clock.

Sometimes females don't want a man to be their nursing assistant. I fully understand that because they have that right.

The first time I walked in and provided care to a lady, she said, "Hell, no, no, no, no. Who is this guy? I don't want him watching me."

On that first day, I got as many residents as I could up for breakfast. Out of thirteen people assigned to me, I was able to get eight up and into the dining room. You don't have time to go by the book. You have to find some shortcuts. Without shortcuts, you can't work as a CNA. It's impossible. I am sure the managers and the CEOs know this.

Once I was able to get patients into the dining room, I had to go back and feed those who were still in bed and unable to get up. Some people eat very well but others are challenged because they don't want to open their mouths to eat. In a lot of cases, the dietitians monitor intake and output. We end up having to put information on the carts that is in a lot of cases not true. The dietician would say, "How much did Mrs. Johnson eat?" And you don't want to say Mrs. Johnson only ate 5 percent. I know situations where people would say, "She ate 50 percent." But in reality, Mrs. Johnson only ate maybe 5 percent. You are just trying to get through the day and if you told the truth, the dieticians would flip out and make you go back and try to get the patient to eat more. But you wouldn't have the time for that.

It's all about time and staffing. The timing and staffing are the heartbeats of good care but often there just isn't enough of either.

That first day I was on my own, running back and forth, making sure the patients are fed. About 90 percent of them are incontinent and they're wet. So you have to attend to them as well. Your coworkers are also busy so they can't help.

I THOUGHT OF QUITTING ON THE FIRST DAY

I THOUGHT ABOUT QUITTING THAT FIRST DAY. MY BACK hurt and so did my mind. You are working for eight hours, but you only get to sit and eat something for thirty minutes. And by the time you walk down to the cafeteria and put your food in the microwave, you probably only have twenty minutes left.

When I left work that first day and went to my car, my entire body was in pain. I had cramps basically all over. It was almost worse than working on a construction site. Mentally and physically, it was exhausting. I think it is one of the most difficult jobs on the planet.

I asked myself, "Should I go back? This is too much." I know people who never went back after orientation.

But when you have a responsibility, you adapt and overcome. You get used to it. You just go in and do it. But there are consequences emotionally and mentally and consequences for the residents and patients as well.

This is a business of shortcuts. And it leads to the question: "Are short-cuts beneficial to the well-being of residents and what we expect as good quality care?" And the answer is no.

My first day on my own was nerve-wracking. Physically, it was more challenging than going to a gym. I remember after my first shift was over, I went to my car and was having muscle contractions. I felt an involuntary movement of muscles in my foot, in my hands, and especially in my stomach. Then I went back the next day and it was not any easier, but the body adapts. I went ahead and just kept doing that. I got used to it and my coworkers started to teach me the real ropes of how to do shortcuts, what you need to do to get through the day because, and at the end of the day, you have to save yourself. You have to save your job and you have to save your body.

In the meantime, you try to do as good a job for the residents as you can. Residents are supposed to walk regularly. They're supposed to do a range of motions. They're supposed to get hydration. So you bring them water at certain times. You try your best to do that, but it's not easy to always remember to do that or even get it done.

On top of all the physical exertion, you also have a lot of paperwork to do. They have a kiosk on the wall, and now they want you to enter a bunch of information about each patient, like their moods and how much they ate. You have to enter that into a computer. You have thirteen people and you have to enter the data for all of them in addition to all the other jobs you have to do—all within the eight-hour shift that you are there for.

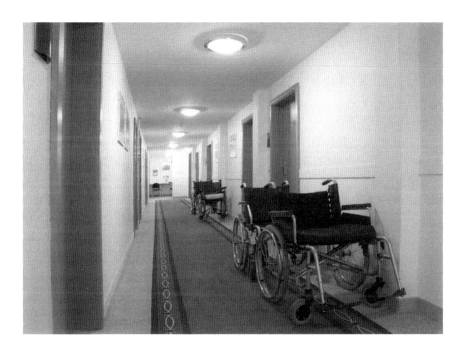

FUN MOMENTS

BUT THERE ARE BRIGHT SPOTS. YOU DO HAVE SOME residents who are funny. The ones who are alert say things that make you laugh and those are the kinds of good points in the day because you get to laugh. I love when a resident is funny and I even kind of like it when residents curse you out.

Cursing you out allows residents to express themselves. I remember this gentleman who was one of the old-time Mafia types, a real street guy from the 1930s or 1940s, and he would still repeat the way he talked to other gang members. He still thought he was living in that time. When you went to his room and you tried to touch him, he would tell you, "You're gonna swim with the fishes," or "You're going to be dead. They're going to find you in the river." He would just go on and on. So that was funny.

But when you fed him, he would be so nice to you. He would say, "You are so good to me. You're my son. You're a nice guy." All of that stuff is extremely funny.

You run into so many different characters. Some of my residents were scientists, microbiologists, former CIA officers, police officers, military officers—from every career you can think of. These are well-accomplished, well-educated, and big people of their times.

I literally learned how to speak the Italian language just from being around different residents.

They tell stories about their lives. They make jokes.

I sometimes wear a turban. Residents sometimes make fun of me for that, asking me if I keep my money in the turban.

They are funny residents, coming from different cultures with different types of jokes.

I remember once I was taking a resident, a nice Italian lady, to the dining room for dinner. I noticed she was looking at my hands. Then she started brushing my hands like she was cleaning something. She looked at me and said, "Don't worry, son, one day we will all be white."

She was making a racial joke but I wasn't offended. I almost died laughing. At her age, she probably had predementia or Alzheimer's. I took her statement as meaning that she wanted good to come for everybody. She wanted all people to be treated fair and equally. That was her way of expressing that. It was a teachable moment as far as her humanity. No matter how people are raised, they still have a soul and good intentions.

You learn so much from residents that you start to feel that you need to do more with your own life. You just see these people who went to college or had big jobs and you look at yourself and start to think that you could do better.

Another fun point in this career is at Christmas. I worked at one facility where every staff member received an envelope. The residents would pick a staff member that they really appreciated and give them sixty dollars, maybe hundred dollars, and put it in a Christmas card to show their appreciation. Families would bring in food, cakes, or they would order catered food. The good facilities spend a lot of money on Christmas parties. A couple of facilities would rent out a banquet room at a Hilton hotel. Staff would dress up. They would have a DJ, food, music, dance, a lot of gifts, and money.

These were privately owned facilities, and they would really go all out.

I have also worked for facilities owned by larger corporations that would do nothing at the end of the year for their employees. They don't even allow their residents to give gifts to staff.

BEING A MALE NURSING ASSISTANT

I GOT USED TO WORKING IN NURSING HOMES. BUT ONE of the challenges that you face as a male nursing assistant, everybody is asking, "Where is the man?"

It is a female-dominated business. A female was your boss. A female was your senior. A female would run it. Male nursing assistants are abused. They think because you're a man, you're strong. You always get the toughest assignments.

They constantly called you to lift. They would give you the heaviest people and sometimes you had to lift people who had tracheostomies and were bedridden. You had to get them up in a recliner with the trach machine so they could breathe.

Everybody is on break, except you. Everybody would get their lunch break, but for males, the work was never done.

If you say no to them, they will talk and gossip about you and call you lazy.

As a man, you really would have to know the psychology of working around a female. You really would have to know when to talk and when not to, when to brush things off, and when to ignore people. I love my mother and I love women. Women are the foundation of life. Working with them as a nursing assistant, you had to have special skills to survive it. And it's also based on their culture, level of education, personality, and emotions.

Male caregivers also are subjected to sexual harassment. Personally, it doesn't bother me. As a man, I don't have a problem with it.

A lot goes on, sexually, in care homes. These are human beings with different situations, feelings, and emotions. I have experienced touching, grabbing. I've had women trying to press their chest against me. I had one supervisor who sat in my lap.

I had a director of nursing who repeatedly called me to her office to massage her back. She would page me on the PA system. When I arrived, she would close the door. Staff would wonder what was going on. When I massaged her back, her shirt would be open. I was behind her. She had very firm breasts. They looked good. I am massaging her back and looking down her shirt and the staff outside is wondering what is going on. I am a hot-blooded male from the Caribbean. It's only natural that I was turned on by this. I'm not a monk and I am not a saint.

She kept doing this until the staff reported her and she was fired.

I've had many different relationships with staff members. I've had one relationship that lasted five years. I've had one-night stands. These were women who were married or in relationships. I've had husbands and boyfriends who would show up at the job, text me, or call. There have been close calls with dangerous people hanging out in parking lots.

These relationships have also ended up in disasters for me. When the relationship is ending, the entire building knows; the females gossip about it. I had a fight one time with my supervisor, in which I dumped a bucket of ice on the floor. All kinds of things happen when you are a male caregiver.

These all happened in the 1990s or early 2000s. Things are much better now with more controls.

Sometimes, when a woman made a remark to me, I just got very quiet. It was the best thing. And when they said something off-color or said something weird, I would say, "Whatever." I was very good at that.

If you were single, you got better treatment. If you were single, at least, you were on the market, and they would be nice to you if you looked good.

I've seen guys come to work dressed like they are going to a party. They are well-groomed because when they come to work, it's all about the girls.

A lot of stuff happened. There was a lot of cheating. Many marriages were ruined. Often, the females aren't home much. They are working double shifts. They get close to males at work and because they are human beings, they end up having relationships. They spend more time with males at work than they do with their husbands.

THE HOUSEKEEPING AND ENVIRONMENTAL DEPARTMENT

ONE OF THE MOST IMPORTANT DEPARTMENTS IN A nursing home is housekeeping/environmental service. In every job, I really would pay a lot of attention to this department.

First, I must say people that work in housekeeping or environmental services are extremely underpaid. They get no respect. Often, they don't have health benefits because they outsource the services to external companies who pay extremely cheap, around seven to eight dollars per hour.

I've seen people from Mexico, Peru, and other Spanish-speaking countries. They can't speak English, so they get jobs at the bottom of the barrel. Sometimes they have criminal records. Sometimes they are transitioning from poverty. They are not people with good work histories or with good educations.

People quit every day. They want more money, so people quit. I've seen people who are only there two weeks before they quit.

One of the things that's hard on them is the chemicals that they breathe every day. They have to use all these sprays, and I see where they're not advised to wear respirators or masks. They spray all these chemicals every day, especially when they're stripping the floor with a buffing machine. It's a big machine and they have to strip the floor and they use certain solutions and chemicals that have a very strong and powerful smell.

When I walk past it, I have a headache, and these people work closely in it every day. I see these people who left their home countries just like I did to come here, and they work like dogs to survive.

I've seen where a door is ripped off of a closet where they keep cleaning solutions, sanitizers, and equipment. It has not been fixed for months. They blame the caregiver for not reporting something that has been going on for months. If maintenance was doing their rounds, they would be able to see that and take care of it.

It just boils down to money. People are hired and a few weeks later, they disappear because they are either not treated respectfully or are underpaid.

THE JOB DESCRIPTION HAS TO BE CLEAR

ONE PROBLEM IN NURSING HOMES IS THAT OFTEN JOB descriptions aren't clear and that allows everybody to pass the buck. Residents frequently go the bathroom on the floor. The housekeepers, with all they're going through, don't want to clean feces off the floor. And then the CNAs feel like it's not their job to do it either. But it's got to be done. There's a stalemate.

I've seen residents throw up and there's blood on the floor. There are different procedures in cleaning up blood, vomit, feces, and other bodily fluids. The CNA, in an ideal situation, would take up the waste material off the ground, and then housekeeping would clean after that. In environmental services, they do the best with what they have.

My problem is with the owners of these places. I really feel bad for the workers and what they have to do given their low pay and benefits. Some of them don't even get health insurance.

Housekeepers are hardworking people with very few resources. These are the people that are on the front line against bacteria and cross-contamination. These people are really important to make sure doorknobs and walls or wherever people are touching are fairly clean and sanitized.

They make sure the place is well-dusted so people with respiratory issues aren't affected. But their job is so extremely important. Without them, I think the residents wouldn't be able to survive as far as bacteria and a clean and safe environment.

THE LAUNDRY
DEPARTMENT

ANOTHER CRUCIAL DEPARTMENT IS THE LAUNDRY.
Facilities are doing everything they can to save money and cut costs by having employees do jobs that are not in their job descriptions. One thing I have seen in laundries is that the facility would buy the machine new and run them for many, many years until they start making loud noises or the motor would burn out. Sometimes you would smell rubber burning. At one facility, the machine made a loud banging sound. These are multi-million-dollar businesses. I worked for one company that has facilities all the way in Germany. But they run washing machines into the ground. The caregivers need to be creative in doing whatever they have to do to get the laundry done.

It's all about the money. But what they don't understand is that it affects the residents and the workers. It increases burnout. They used to have people in the housekeeping department who would stop by the resident's room and pick up their laundry, wash the clothes, fold them, and bring them back. Now, they are overwhelming the caregivers with the extra work of bringing the laundry to the laundry and washing the clothes themselves when the caretakers have so much other work to do.

It causes lots of problems. The machines aren't working well. Caregivers are so busy that they have no time to go by the book and clothes are lost. I have seen caregivers, when the dryers are not working properly, hang up clothes in the closet that are soaking wet. That doesn't mean that they are bad workers. They are just overwhelmed, overworked, and underpaid. Sometimes you will have three of four residents with laundry and if the dryer is not working properly, you have to go back and forth. No one has that kind of time. You may have nine or ten residents who need laundry, showers. With a machine that does not work, it's only normal. It goes back to funding and not necessarily anything the workers are doing wrong. At the end of the day, the owners sit back and make money by cutting budgets. The families need to be much more involved if they care about their loved ones.

Smart family members take the resident's clothes home, wash it, fold it, and bring it back. I'm not suggesting that this is easy for all family members.

Some places are very good at tracking residents' or patients' clothing, and some are not. With the laundry, everybody has to play their part. In some facilities, all clothes are washed at one time. If clothes are not labeled, you will never be able to match the clothing with the resident. It just disappears in the midst of the laundry department.

The clothes should be labeled, and family members can help with that. But it doesn't always work out that way.

People who work in the laundry department maybe get paid little bit more than those in other departments, but they also work very hard. I have noticed more owners outsourcing both environmental services and the laundry departments as a way to cut costs.

The facility where I currently work has an effective laundry system. They wash the clothes individually and bring them back personally and put them up in the residents' room. The same person who washed the clothes, folds the laundry, and brings it back to the residents' room. That is how it should be, but sadly, most facilities don't make the effort because it takes more time and money to do it the right way.

I have noticed that laundry workers are usually older employees closer to retirement. No young person would ever work in the laundry. I have seen some facilities that even resort to going to laundry mats. Maybe it's cheaper for them to do that. It all boils down to the math, the amount of money the facility has to spend.

THE MAINTENANCE
DEPARTMENT

THE MAINTENANCE DEPARTMENT IS A DIFFERENT STORY
because these guys have a lot of experience and are paid well. They have a
very important job to keep the building functioning. From my experience,
most maintenance departments are very efficient. I've also seen the flip side of
that—maintenance that doesn't get to issues for weeks, which affects the residents greatly. For example, a bed that won't decline. I've seen where residents
have to eat or drink and just are barely reclined because the bed doesn't work.

That could lead to other health issues if someone is not able to sit properly when they are eating. Wheelchairs also often have problems with the
brakes or wheels. Maintenance people get to it as soon as they can. But
it depends on their workload and in some cases, it can take weeks to fix
the issue.

Heating and cooling are often an issue. I've seen where temperatures are
too cold, and it takes a while for them to fix it. And I have seen temperatures
that are too hot. So, maintenance is nonstop.

Fire drills are important since we are dealing with so many different
chemicals. There have been quite a few nursing facilities that have burned
down. Some companies are very good at having fire drills and educating
employees about what to do in case of a fire. There's a lot to learn and a lot
to know about fires.

For example, you have to know which residents to move out first. You do
not take the elevator; you take the stairs. You can use sheets to pull people out

who are very heavy. Make sure the doors are closed. You feel the temperature of the door before you open it.

I've seen some nursing facilities that are six-floor high, but fortunately, many of them now are between one and two.

Then you have oxygen in the rooms. You have some residents who smoke. We tell them, "Don't smoke inside, smoke outside." As a CNA, you have to be vigilant and watch everything.

One area that the maintenance department oversees is clearing out patient rooms once the resident dies.

They are often faced with the decision of whether to throw out items in a dumpster or asking a staff member if they them. In 90 percent of the case, there are items that are in good shape, such as an expensive leather chair. If a resident can afford to pay the cost of assisted living, in a lot of cases, they can also afford quality, name-brand products.

I've seen staff members get fifty- to sixty-inch televisions that would otherwise have been tossed in the dumpster.

One lady owned a big mansion on the Jersey Shore. She had so much money she didn't know what to do with it all. When she died, most of her furniture was given away to staff members. For staff that can't afford luxury items, that's a good thing.

At the same time, I have seen very expensive medical equipment such as wheelchairs and walkers, breathing equipment just dumped in the garbage. That is a shame. It also sends a message that no matter what you own, at the end of your time, none of these objects can help you. As the saying goes, "You can't take it with you."

THE RECREATION DEPARTMENT

I HAVE A LOT OF RESPECT FOR THE RECREATION department. So far in my career, I haven't seen anything negative about this department in most facilities. Recreation helps residents with memory, balance, and it gives them mental stimulation. I'm not an expert on what recreation does, but I know it gives them a bit of joy. They play different games with them. They play music from back in their time, such as Frank Sinatra. They bring back the memories from back in those days, and I see that it stimulates them a lot. They take residents shopping. At the end of the day, it's more than just feeding someone and putting clothes in them. Mental stimulation is important. I see the big improvements this makes with the residents and how they react.

I see residents who are upset and nothing you can do will calm them down. But as soon as you put on a Tony Bennett record, it brings them back to that time when they were happy and they are reliving it. Music—as I am a musical person myself—is one of the most powerful things.

The other department that does a lot of good for residents is the beauty salon. It helps residents to feel young and vibrant. You can feel the energy after they come out of the beauty salon. I see that and I feel good about it because the residents are happy. They walk differently, they feel different, and all these people say to them, "Wow, you look so nice." So, within the context of all that's going on, I think it's a very good thing.

THE PHYSICAL THERAPY DEPARTMENT

THE OTHER DEPARTMENT THAT REALLY HELPS RESI-dents is the physical therapy department. It gives residents their strength back, which helps with mobility and range of motion. It helps with their mental health as well. Anyone that brings anything positive to the residents as far as stimulation, I give them credit.

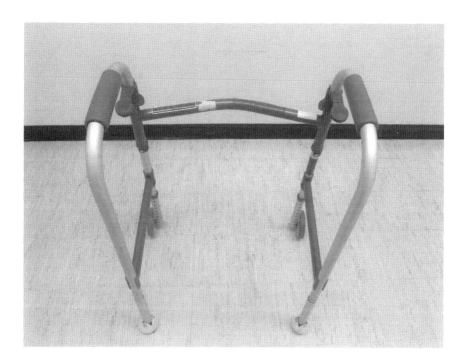

ADAPT AND OVERCOME

OVER THE YEARS, YOU ADAPT TO THE LIFE OF A CNA and you overcome. Your body adapts naturally to working in that environment. You develop a rhythm in how to function every day, and basically, you go into survival mode. You must follow the policy. You must follow the laws. You must follow the rules.

But as a worker who is overwhelmed—who is bombarded unrealistically with workloads—you have to find a way to survive, to keep your job and provide good care to the residents. It's a very weird balance. It's not an easy balance. So, to survive the eight hours that you're working and wanting that person and that resident or patient to feel comfortable, safe and warm—and for you to still have your back strong and to do another shift—you have to take shortcuts.

There's a disconnect between government policies as it relates to patients' or residents' care and the owner's interest. The only person who actually cares is the actual caregiver.

There are family members, of course. I would never sit here and generalize and say, "Family members don't care about their loved ones." But from my experience, a lot of them don't. I used the phrase "a lot," not all.

When you walk into these facilities, everything looks good. If you're a visitor and you see everybody in their wheelchairs and you hear people singing and clapping, of course, that looks good. However, you don't see when one of these people has to go to the bathroom, but can't stand up. There's always someone who will say, "We will be with you in a minute." That minute maybe turns out to be an hour. It's not because the caregiver can't help, but the caregiver is so busy. They're making beds really fast, trying to change linens, or maybe assist other residents who are bedridden such as those with tracheotomies and have to be turned or those who have bed sores.

You cannot always stop everything to take someone to the toilet. You really have to do what it takes to survive and it's not easy. The people in my industry are very skillful and mentally strong. Most of them do their best with the resources that they have.

THE PANDEMIC

IN EARLY 2020, I HEARD ABOUT A NEW VIRUS THAT WAS sweeping the world. But at that time, we didn't know much about it at first. We just heard about it on the news. In the early days, few people were taking it as seriously as they should have been. We had no idea it was going to reach our doorsteps.

I was in France in early 2020 because I have a child there. Returning to the United States in March of that year on a plane from Paris to Canada, there was a person on the plane sneezing and coughing the entire time. At the time, we didn't know much about the virus, nor did we take it very seriously, particularly health-care workers. We slowly started to react with increased hand washing, that kind of thing. But the precautions in the early spring of 2020 were nowhere near the level of those that we would take later in the pandemic.

Back in the United States, I started working actively again after being abroad for a while. I was shocked to see a lot of sick people, residents dying like flies left to right. Psychologically, it was a big shock.

I started asking about certain residents who were no longer there.

"They died from COVID," I was told.

I was extremely shocked and horrified that people I took care of were dropping like flies.

On one of my first assignments after coming back from Europe, I was assisting a lady who was drooling and dripping mucous, coughing, with a high temperature. I was up in her face as I took care of her. I had a mask on, but COVID-19 was still not something we were too worried about. We still didn't know that the virus was as highly transmissible as it was or as dangerous.

But I caught COVID-19 from this resident.

As more and more residents began to die from COVID-19, the facility where I worked imposed restrictions and safeguards such as using personal protective equipment and isolating infected patients.

Workers were calling in sick. All of a sudden, everything was going crazy.

Then it was my turn. I got sick and had to be out of work for two weeks. Those were the worst two weeks of my life.

I experienced the first symptoms one night working the two-to-nine shift. I was taking care of a resident when I felt a burst of energy. My body was full of energy. I was sweating, like I had just come out of a gym. That only lasted ten to twenty minutes. Then I started having a headache and then I started feeling hot.

"Could you check my temperature, please?" I asked my supervisor.

It was through the roof, close to 102. The supervisor had to report it, mailing the administrator and others. My body felt weird. I started having hot flashes. I left for the emergency room. By the time I arrived, my temperature had dropped to around 99, so the hospital did not want to admit me. But I was forceful, telling them that I had been in Europe and that I had been caring for residents who were positive for COVID-19. I had to keep insisting until they found me a room. A doctor saw me for less than five minutes, listening to my lungs. My COVID was upper respiratory and did not go to my lungs.

It was interesting that I was positive for COVID-19 but the residents I was caring for didn't catch it. These were people in their nineties. Something in their immune system must have protected them. That would make a great subject for a study. That's something scientists need to look at.

I left the hospital and went home. For two weeks, I could not sleep; I could not eat. I was scared to go to sleep because I thought I would never wake up. My temperature was through the roof. I lost a lot of weight.

One of the biggest mistakes I made was to watch the news. I was sick and watching stories about people dropping like flies. I saw stories about people in Italy crying and begging for help from God. In New York, they were putting dead bodies in refrigerated trailers. There were so many of dead bodies that they didn't know where to put them. I was horrified. These were human beings. All of this was traumatic.

I don't like taking medicine, so I was trying natural remedies, boiling orange peels and ginger, taking vitamins.

I could not hold down food, so I had no strength. I could not walk. When I tried to train myself to walk again, I did not have a steady gait. I was rocking back and forth. I would take a few steps and then sit down. I was dizzy all the time.

I live alone so there was no help for me when I was sick. Once I tried to go to the supermarket. I drove to the parking lot but was so weak I could not get out of the car. I had to turn around and drive home.

COVID kills your drive. You feel like you have nothing to live for. You can't accomplish anything. You're just weak.

I took Tylenol for pain and to bring down my temperature. I could eat certain things that I didn't normally eat such as raisin bagels with jelly. I could hold down half of one slice and that was all I ate for an entire day.

I let the virus run its course through my system. Up to this day, a year later, I do not turn the light off when I go to sleep. I don't have any long-lasting effects from COVID. I feel good. I am fully vaccinated now.

After my 14 days of isolation were over, my employer had me meet them in the parking lot to check my temperature. They checked it three times, on three different days, before I could come back to work.

Back at work, it was very tense. All the residents were isolated in their rooms. We had to wear masks, gowns, gloves. Everyone realized now that this was no joke. It wiped out a lot of residents. People were dying, dying, dying. I remember one time in particular, a man named Ludi who was very funny, a very nice guy who was always making us laugh.

Not only physically but mentally it was a very tough time for everyone.

Before the vaccines became available, family members could not even visit. They could make phone calls or video calls or look through the windows at their loved ones. There were people dying with families unable to say goodbye in person. That was very stressful for the residents and their family members.

The physical and mental toll on residents was unbelievable and inconceivable. Most already had health issues before COVID, which is why they were in a nursing home to begin with. Then, to be unable to see their family gave them a sense of isolation. Depression kicks in. Everything snowballed. If they tested positive for COVID, we had to isolate the residents from other residents, further increasing the isolation. They would be locked in their rooms for days, not just a couple of hours. That had to be damaging. They only saw their caretakers and the caretakers were scared of catching COVID themselves. I had to deliver meals and it was almost delivering meals in a jail. You just drop them off, quickly and nervously open stuff for them because and run out. We did not want to stay in a resident's room even for a minute.

Personal hygiene was also a problem. Even with personal protection equipment, the staff was totally paranoid and scared. It was a very, very sad situation.

The caregivers were worried about getting the virus themselves and bringing it home to their spouse and children. I would guess that many residents did not receive personal hygienic care during COVID and certainly not proper care because the caregivers were so nervous. I'm talking about mouth care, body care.

I can't find the words to describe it. It was worse than hell. Staff members felt guilty. We felt bad that we were not able to provide the best care.

Even the workers had to make sure not to get too close to each other. Some people were scared and embarrassed to say whether they had tested positive. Staff members were listening out for the names of people who staying out of work for a week or two. It was hush-hush because at that time people were embarrassed to be known as positive COVID. When people were positive, you only knew because they didn't show up for work. There would be rumors and gossip anytime someone missed a day of work. "Maybe they're positive," people would say. Even though management tried to keep it confidential, it always seemed to come out about who tested positive. I remember that after I returned to work, coworkers would scorn me, just because they were not positive at the time and I had been. They would literally run away from me. I remember one worker who sprayed a disinfectant every time a co-worker who had tested positive walked past her. It was a very strange time. Everyone was acting different. Everyone was acting suspiciously.

Later, the same people who ran away from me and shunned their coworkers tested positive. COVID does not discriminate. Anybody can get it, prime ministers, kings, queens. All of us.

At first, management was being very stingy with personal protective equipment. There were staff members who were stealing it and taking it home. So eventually, they were issuing PPE only on demand. But later on, we had enough.

Making matters worse, we had a lot of staff members calling in sick so there was a severe shortage of staff. Those of us who were healthy earned a lot of overtime pay.

We as health care workers were scared. We had to care for patients who were positive and that often involves coming in close contact with them. Who wants to wash the face of someone who has COVID? We were on the frontlines, working around a virus that could literally kill us. Yet most of us got up out of bed and came to work every day, putting our lives on the line to help other people live.

I remember one resident who had COVID-19 and was recovering. She was about to be taken to a doctor's appointment and was walking through the lobby. She suddenly fell down and went into convulsions, trembling and shaking and dying. I joined two of my coworkers and we started CPR. She had a mask on but when we did compressions, she was still blowing out air. There were several members of management around, but they hid, scared to help.

The paramedics arrived, but we lost her.

As health-care workers, I believe, we did more than our share during COVID-19 pandemic.

It was stressful in part because the restrictions were constantly changing. Sometimes they were strict and then they would be loosened. We would be required to frequently test residents sometimes, and then later those requirements would be lifted and then come back again with the next surge of COVID-19. No funerals were allowed. I saw patients die and go straight from an assisted living facility to cremation with families unable to see their loved ones before they left. It had a severe psychological effect on family members. It was brutal on the mind.

It's better now, even though we still have to take precautions with the new variants on the scene. We still have to go through temperature checks and COVID-19 tests every two days. By the time the results are in, it's time to get tested again. You do feel like you are tested every single day. There is mental wear and tear with that. The staff gets really tired of being tested. There are a lot of false positives, particularly with the rapid tests, and that increases the stress. You have to miss work for another fourteen days. They also have to retest everybody in the building and you are not able to pick up work at any other facility either because of the positive test results. There are times when I cleaned my nose out with cotton balls before I was tested because you don't want to miss any more work or any more paychecks. I finally started giving myself the tests because the testers were going deeper and deeper into my nose and down into my throat. So, I started doing the swab myself.

I am weary of this, and I am sure other health workers are as well, especially ICU workers who have to wear suits and respirators. While I was going through all this stress, I lost one of my favorite uncles to COVID-19. He had an underlying condition called sickle cell anemia.

It's very hard. On top of that, you have to deal with the guilt when people you work with die. I don't think people grasp the amount of stress health-care workers endure. They are some of the strongest people I know. Hopefully, society will look back one day on the contribution of health-care workers and appreciate it.

I applaud the federal government for providing funding for assisted living facilities during the pandemic. At the same time, very little of this money made its way down to the front-line workers. If you think about the fact that caregivers are often doing the laundry, maintenance, and other jobs over and above their own, you would think that the facilities would hand out raises or bonuses during COVID-19. Some have but many others haven't.

I have been vaccinated for COVID-19 but some of my coworkers have not and I respect that decision. However, some of the facilities are now requiring workers to be vaccinated, so those who refuse are out and just add more work on the rest of us. I believe facilities are correct in requiring staff to be vaccinated. We are dealing with elderly people. If you want to work in health care, I believe you should be vaccinated.

As I write this, new variants are gaining ground. It is even worse than the earlier variants as far as the rate of transmission. It's more serious than the regular virus, and that says a lot.

Even though I am fully vaccinated, at work, I wear a mask, goggles and other protective equipment. But as I venture out around New Jersey, I see many people not wearing masks even though the delta variant is spreading. When you watch the news, everyone seems to be alert to the new threat. But in the real world, people don't seem to be taking extra precautions to the extent that they should. I see family members coming to the assisted living facility to visit their loved ones and all they do is wear a mask and check their temperature at the door. Yet the delta variant is highly contagious. When I go into a grocery store wearing a mask, people look at me like I'm crazy.

I take the virus seriously. I had it and I know what it feels like. I still have flashbacks and anxiety. I am scared to get it again. I also don't want to pass it on to the residents I care for. One of the things people don't realize is that we are headed into a new world, a new reality. It's not going back to normal. Coronavirus is not going away. We are the ones who are going to have to corona. We don't know how it may mutate. We have to be careful.

I think back to the day I was born and how many vaccinations I have in my body since I was a child. When I look at the COVID-19 vaccine, I see that very few people have dropped dead from getting it. What do I have to lose? I have a son overseas. I have relationships in Ethiopia and France. I travel around the world a lot. It's only common sense to trust the vaccine. It's not like it was years ago when vaccines were used as weapons.

I think COVID-19 is going to have a long-term effect on the psychology of human beings. It is something we have never seen before.

I had serious anxiety about returning to work after I had COVID-19. I was in fear of being infected again. If you combine that stress with all the regular stress that comes with a job and all the things you are seeing and hearing about the virus from around the world, you really start to develop serious anxiety. In many cases, you aren't sleeping well at night anyway because you are worried about COVID-19 pandemic. Then you have to get up in the morning and go to work with people who are positive with the virus.

At the same time, people were politicizing the pandemic for their own benefit, attacking New York Gov. Andrew Cuomo and others for their handling of the crisis. People are crazy. They used the pandemic to benefit themselves. There are people who filed illegal claims.

Some people stayed home from work during COVID-19 while we came to work every day, and now they want to come back. I think most organizations and companies manipulated COVID-19 to avoid paying bills. COVID-19 is a bad virus and did a lot of damage, but human beings also manipulate and abuse COVID-19 for their own benefit, even to this day. There was a time during the pandemic that nursing homes could not do any new admissions. I'm sure that hurt their profits a little bit but these people make so much money that I'm sure they didn't feel it.

The government tried to use COVID-19 to control people.

COVID-19 did affect every fiber of our lives, psychologically, physically, financially. It brought out a lot about the true quality of human beings. It exposed a lot about the narcissistic and greedy nature of some people.

I will say that since I was unable to travel during COVID-19 and I worked a lot of overtime, my life actually improved during the pandemic.

It gave me time to clean up my financial life and make sure my credit was good and I saved some money. It prompted me to think about buying my first house, maybe back in Jamaica. It gave me a chance to refocus and reset my life. COVID-19 was terrible but there were some positive aspects of it as well, as strange as that may seem. You saw true colors, in people, in families, in companies, in kids.

It provided clarity into the human condition.

The pandemic is in its third year. Cases dropped, but came surging back in late 2021 and early 2022. Staff members are once again being tested so frequently that we feel like we're back in 2020. But it's not nearly as bad as it was back then.

Many of the residents who were vaccinated are not testing positive again, fortunately. But others, including staff members, who were vaccinated are testing positive. So now the talk is booster shots. There are a lot of staff members who don't want a third shot.

The pandemic wears you down psychologically. There is one facility where I go to pick up extra hours. The administrator told me I was not allowed to work there, at least temporarily, because more than 20 percent of the residents and staff had tested positive for COVID-19. This is a fully vaccinated facility. So, two years out, COVID-19 is still with us. I have coworkers who had the virus who complain that they lost their sense of taste. For me, it's 90 percent better than it was, but still lingering. In some facilities, workers who test positive are having to use their earned sick leave during quarantine. That's the only way they can get paid. These are employees who are literally risking their lives by coming to work to care for patients who can infect them with a potentially deadly virus, and they are having to use their sick leave after they test positive. At the same time, these facilities are getting government COVID-19 assistance- taxpayer dollars – during the pandemic. At one point early on in the pandemic, facilities were giving employees extra hazard pay, but that stopped long ago.

Luckily, I haven't got sick after having COVID-19 and two doses of the vaccine. So far, so good. But you never know when you work around a lot of overtime and your body is tired and run down. You never know what will make you get sick. I still haven't decided whether I will take a booster shot.

I don't think we will ever completely avoid COVID-19. Relatives come into facilities to visit, and we don't know if they are positive or not or whom they have been exposed to. All the facilities do is a temperature check. They walk in off the street, take a temperature check, and then start mingling with the residents. It's a repetitive cycle. The facilities don't want to offend the relatives—who after all are paying the bill—so they allow them to come in with only a temperature check and not proof of a negative test.

So I think COVID-19 will be with us for a long time. I suppose we have to keep on taking booster shots. But how many will be enough?

Meanwhile, COVID-19 continues to affect every aspect of assisted living and geriatrics in general. There is a worker shortage, even in the dietary department. The facilities are desperate for people to work and they can't find staff. The shortage of staff causes issues in every aspect of the quality of care. Sometimes it bothers me to see caregivers risking their lives to come work every day and the owners—who are taking no health risks—earning ten times more than the caregivers.

Once there was a situation when one of my patients went into convulsions and was literally dying. I was administering CPR along with two of my coworkers. With each compression, the patient was literally breathing in our faces.

The administrator and the registered nurse were standing behind a wall just watching us, unwilling to help.

We are taking risks every day at work while people who have paid massive amounts of money are not taking any. It's sad. You try to find some humanity but it's very difficult to find.

It seems as if there is no end to the COVID-19. It is a nightmare, but a repetitive nightmare from which you never wake up. Most of the staff who have been vaccinated and received their booster shots, have now tested positive for COVID-19. Even the human resources director at the company where I currently work tested positive three or four times, despite being vaccinated and boosted. It affects staffing because people can't come to work if they test positive.

The same happened to my manager. But far fewer residents are not dying this time from COVID-19. Other than that, everything seems the same.

We have family members walking in off the streets to visit their relatives and all they are doing is checking their temperatures. They are not testing them for COVID-19. Someone who is asymptomatic could walk in and never be noticed. It's a nonstop cycle.

MONEY TREES

IT'S SAD TO SAY, BUT IN MANY FACILITIES, PATIENTS are like money trees to the owners.

All types of therapists and other health-care providers are constantly streaming through the facilities. That includes lab technicians performing tests.

I acknowledge that some testing, some therapy, can be important and necessary for residents. If family members request it, that's one thing. But in many cases, facilities are just ordering the therapy and the tests for no other reason than for the money they get from the residents or their families. It's a way to generate cash.

In some cases, speech therapy and physical therapy are necessary and if the resident can afford it, it can help them live better lives in their final years.

But I have seen therapists come into a facility and engage the staff members in long conversations about their personal lives. I'm not exactly sure how they are being paid. If it is by the hour then much of the time is not spent on the patient but on small talk. I noticed that one therapist would come for about forty-five minutes. She would spend a few minutes with the patient, make a few notes, and spend the rest of the time talking to staff members about her personal life.

The patient, by the way, was a gentleman who was in a state of decline with age. He was slowly losing his memory, but he was still able to feed himself and he was eating. I am not suggesting that therapy wouldn't help. But in many cases, I'm not sure why the therapists are there other than to make money for themselves and the facility. Everybody seems to be making money all the way through the resident's last days.

Sometimes residents will stop eating simply because they don't like the food or the temperature of the food. They don't like cold sandwiches at every meal. But the facility will call in a therapist who spends most of their time having conversations with the staff about unrelated topics. How does this make sense? It seems to me like a big waste of money to me.

Physical therapy is important, of course. But I also think it can be abused. I worked at a facility once where the physical therapy department billed for treatments that were either not done, were not effective, or were nonsensical. They use equipment that doesn't improve the patient's condition. They use heavy braces that don't help therapeutically. These things are not free.

In some cases, the therapists don't explain to the staff how to properly use the braces. If a staff member is not there when the therapist puts a brace on, they may either leave it off or put it on incorrectly. But the patient is still being charged for it. A lot of the equipment is actually being rented.

My point is that there are so many ways to make money off residents. The therapists in many cases are unsupervised, unregulated. They can just write something down on a piece of paper that says the patient needs therapy even if they don't. They do so much unnecessary treatment and everybody is making money off this.

Even treatment that is necessary could have been avoided if the resident had been properly cared for in the first place. For example, when you have a resident who slides out of a chair after sitting on that chair for eight to ten hours, that is an issue of inadequate care. Facilities may not have the staff to properly attend to the residents. Many facilities will only hire extra staff if they absolutely are forced to do so.

In many cases, residents are like children who need total care and attention. They can't speak or turn themselves or do anything independently. They are placed in institutions without the staffing to take care of all those needs. So, you will have a lot of breakdowns in the care.

At the same time, money is there to be made at every step of the way. Even psychiatry is in on it. I've seen psychiatrists come in because they told a resident had a mental issue such as depression. Sometimes depression is caused by a physical, not mental, condition. Someone could have a urinary tract infection and a psychiatrist is called in. The resident is crying out for help but can't verbalize their needs. The psychiatrist will sit there and write pages and pages of notes and then, of course, sends a bill.

I am sure there are many cases where psychiatrists help patients. But in a general facility where patients don't have a history of mental health issues, they are often misdiagnosed and then must pay for the bill.

This is the world they are placed in. They are not in a world where people are going to shower them with love, necessarily. Sure, there is *some* humanity. But still, the residents are in a for-profit universe. That universe is there to make a profit.

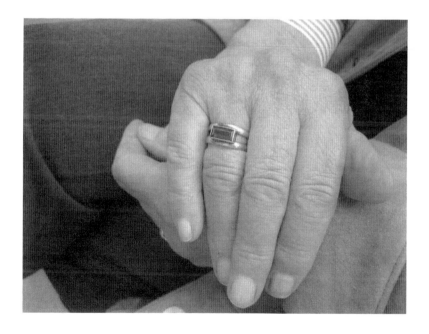

OPERATING UNDER AN ILLUSION

A LOT OF THE RESIDENTS ARE UNDER THE ILLUSION that this will not be permanent. They think it will just be temporary. A lot of them are hoping that one day, they're going to leave. If they're developing Alzheimer's or dementia, it's easy for them to feel that way. But someone who doesn't have any mental issues realizes, "This is it for me and my kids have no time to take care of me."

Some of them adapt to it very well. They say, "This is my reality. I'm not leaving. I'm not going anywhere. My kids can't take care of me if I fall or if I have to use the bathroom."

But there is often a disconnect between family members and residents. I have seen family members act as if they don't even know how to touch their own family members when something goes wrong.

They say, "Oh my God, can you come? She's coughing and she needs a tissue. I don't know what to do." The natural instinct would be to get involved if you really loved your family member.

All too often, they look at the elderly as just someone who is weak. But they also are human beings with some emotions and feelings. They get depressed because they're not able to control their bowels, they're not able to do things and they're losing all their power, their friends, and their families. That depression further deteriorates the body. We're social beings and when we are isolated psychologically, we are being drained and we're dying. That's a big problem.

The Disruption of Sudden Changes

By the time most residents end up in an assisted living center, they have probably lived for decades with their spouse, often in the same home or neighborhood. They have become accustomed to doing things in a certain way. They eat each night at the dinner table, spending time with their families. Then, all of a sudden, everything changes when they reach a certain age. It has a psychological effect when they are suddenly given orders on when to eat, when to take a shower, when to go to bed. It is traumatic when they lose their independence, especially when you add the impact of medication and health problems. It's a scary scenario when you lose control over everything in your life. I often wonder if family members are under the effects of losing power. That's why I think getting old is scary. One of the worst things a person can go through is to have nothing to look forward to. They can't make plans. They lose a sense of hope. All of this is traumatic, which is why it's important for family members to be more patient with their elderly relatives as they transition into this new world. It's definitely not easy.

They are like lost souls. They walk around asking for their family, asking for their lives. They are still alert, still cognizant. They're not stupid. You might tell them their kids are coming tomorrow, their car is outside. They keep searching for their families. Staff members are trained in how to deal with this. But in many cases, we have to lie to them. But they know you are lying to them. They know something is wrong. So they keep asking, searching, wanting to go home. It can be a nightmare scenario. For the residents, it's living hell.

It's one thing if you have full-blown dementia. You are not aware in those cases. You don't remember family or your past life. These patients can live day by day without worrying. But those who are not fully gone and are still alert *do* worry. They fret. They are stressed about everything. I only talk about this so that the readers can understand the transition the residents go through.

I was once working in South Jersey and there was a newly admitted resident. She stopped me and asked, "Sir, where is this place? Where am I?"

I started to explain to her the best I could where the facility was located. She was totally shocked. She wanted to know why she was there. She wanted to know where her kids were.

"Is this a bad dream?" she asked me. "Is this a nightmare?"

She could still remember everything about her house, her kid's names—everything a normal person could remember. But now she is in a place where she knows no one. There was no one on staff to do a one-on-one talk about this. One would expect a family member would have briefed her. I assume they did but it did not register long-term and now she was lost. She was crying profusely, asking, "Where is my family? Did my family abandon me?"

Then she started packing her clothes to leave. But the doors are bolted and locked. All one has to do is put themselves in this scenario to understand what it's like when your life is taken away and you are locked up. No one intentionally does this to be cruel. It's just the transition from being a functional, independent human being to someone who is dependent on other people for everything, and you still have cognitive abilities.

Getting old is no joke. This resident had been a teacher. She had a well-accomplished life and now was down to nothing, eating food that is in many cases not nutritious, and being told what to do. Is this what a normal society should do? Other societies that have nothing in terms of money or material wealth don't do this. Old people are still in control and they have family members around them and are still able to make decisions.

"Ian, do not get old," many residents have advised me.

Something to Think About

In my experience of living in Jamaica and traveling around the world, I had never heard of Alzheimer's disease or dementia until I came to the United States. I never saw it in the elderly in my home country. Maybe we just didn't recognize it. In Jamaica and other parts of the Caribbean, many older residents—I won't say all—go through the phases of their lives with all their cognitive abilities intact. Even In South America and the poorer countries of Cuba and Haiti, you don't see or even hear of many signs of dementia and

Alzheimer's. That's not to say that there isn't some loss of mental ability later in life. But it begs the question of whether Alzheimer's and dementia are a normal part of aging.

I lived in Ethiopia for six years. I have traveled all over Europe. I've just never seen this phenomenon in the elderly that we have in the United States.

I have no evidence that it is unique to the U.S. I am not a doctor or a researcher. But I do work in the field, on the front lines, so to speak, and I travel a lot as well. So I get to see things from both perspectives, hands-on and globally.

When I was in Italy for three years, I saw people in their eighties and nineties outside farming. Italian females in particular seem to have all of their faculties well into later life. The same is true in Ethiopia. I've seen really old people who are still able to communicate and function. In fact, in Ethiopia and most of Africa, nursing homes don't even exist.

I'm not sure what it is. But it's shockingly curious. Is it diet? Is it the environment? Water?

The fact that I live in the United States makes me even more curious because I would like to protect myself from whatever factors may be the cause.

If you think about the fact that Americans are the most medicated people on the planet, yet they also have the highest number of Alzheimer's and dementia in the world, it makes you wonder what is happening here. It begs a lot of questions. Does medication somehow affect the brain? Does the residue of the medication end up in our water? Could it be the preservatives in our food? I just don't know but I feel compelled to ask the question.

If it is true that the numbers are higher here, that's a real issue that needs to be addressed.

Perhaps it is a side effect of being one of the richest countries in the world. I can tell you that about half of the foods that are available in the U.S. are not available in France. You also don't see food packed with preservatives in France. The French seem to be more conservative with additives. I don't find peanut butter in France. Or macaroni and cheese. Maybe they exist but you don't see them as commonly as you do in the United States.

The countries that have fewer choices in foods and that have more organic food seem to have less Alzheimer's dementia.

Lifestyle could also be a factor. In many countries, people walk. They ride bikes. In Europe, almost everyone rides a bike. In Africa, even fewer people have cars.

In the United States, the wider availability of products, stimulants, preservatives, and chemicals is a big business. It could make Alzheimer's and dementia worse.

It could also be stress. With wealth, there is a lot of stress. When you have a society where everyone is overmedicated, stressed out, exposed to toxic chemicals, you will have a higher number of people with dementia. I can say that with confidence, and I welcome someone to prove me wrong.

The pharmaceutical companies must know this. The government must know this. It's a for-profit cycle. The pharmaceutical companies will be the ones who profit the most from medications that will treat dementia. They are not interested in natural remedies or changing lifestyles because they wouldn't benefit financially from those solutions.

Admissions, Sales, and Marketing

These are the employees who come up with the voice mail messages that make assisted living centers sound like heaven. They are the people that try to recruit residents to the facilities. They are well-trained in what to say, how to say it, the smiles, kissing butts, whatever they have to do to get you in. They have an agenda, they have goals, and they know what and whom they are looking for.

They find out what your budget is and the more money you can pay, the harder they will recruit you to live in their facility. They will promise you everything. They are well-dressed, in suit and tie, smiling constantly. The way they look and walk around is impressive, just like the outside of the facility might look good, but inside not so much. They put a lot of money into the face of the facility, beautification with flowers and landscaping and all that. You walk up and you look at the building and it looks great. The sales and marketing are like a dog. When a potential new client walks in, they look happy, almost like they were trained to play the part, and they probably were. The family members are dog lovers and they're ready for a rubbing. It's a psychological condition. It's not that it's bad or evil but it is amazing. Coming from a different culture, I've never seen anything like that. But they do a very good job of getting you to put your relative in the assisted living center. Up to fifteen thousand dollars per month per patient is no joke. It's big money so they do everything they can initially to get residents in.

It's a cat-and-mouse game with sales and marketing. I've seen sales directors do the math. It's like they have a split personality, one if the numbers work out, another if they do not. They don't like it if the residents' families pay attention to details or ask a lot of questions. They don't like it either if the residents' family ask for a tour or an inspection. Some families insist on a tour, checking for smells. Salespeople don't like this.

What they will do to counteract this is announce a tour for prospective clients on a certain date. They will tell the staff so that they can do extra cleaning up, fixing up of the place.

I remember one tour that came through. The residents were relaxing, watching television. But the staff members were putting on a nice performance. The women from the recreation department had their tambourines, all their games. They were singing, clapping, dancing, doing everything for that few minutes during the tour. The staff member who hosted the tour greeted all of us by name. It was a nice act, an Academy Award–winning performance to impress the family members. As soon as they left, we went right back to normal. The smiles and the friendly hellos faded. We all went along with it because the person who is signing your paycheck expects you to. If this was the norm, there would be no need to put on an act. Trust me, this is not the norm. I have worked at some good facilities. But in most, they only put out 100 percent effort when they have a tour coming through.

At the end of the day, it's about the money. They know how much money you have and how much you will have left when you die—if you have any left.

In the beginning, they promise you physical therapy, nice meals, everything. But I can tell you with 100 percent certainty, they never come close to delivering all that.

I remember one resident's daughter who performed a serious inspection. She looked; she smelled; she did everything. She was very upset with some of the things she saw. The admissions director was getting aggravated and pissed off, not in front of the residents, but she was very angry that the woman was so picky. The woman left and the admissions director was bad-mouthing her. "We don't want her in here anyway," she said of the woman's mother.

It's an ugly side of the business. Raising expectations to get your business and then failing to deliver.

The historical socio-economical divide

I have noticed that historically, there are two different worlds in the United States in terms of assisted living. Even though we are all living in the same economy, there is a cultural divide.

People of African and Asian descent, historically, have seemed to be more likely to keep their loved ones at home as they get older rather than in a nursing home. They take turns taking care of loved ones. Even if they do put them in facilities, they tend to be more involved, visiting every day.

In assisted living, you hardly see any residents of African descent. This could be because of the high costs. The starting rate in many cases is ten thousand dollars a month at minimum and can go as high as fourteen thousand dollars and higher. That means that 99.9 percent of residents who can afford this are of Caucasian descent. I have maybe seen one or two people of African descent, and they had been well-paid professional people, doctors and lawyers.

The admissions staff in assisted living screen applicants based on their wealth. In order to be eligible for many facilities, you have to have at least

$250,000 in your account. I'm not saying that people of African descent don't have that amount. But in my experience, I haven't come across those cases very often. Also, culturally, we try to keep our family members at home as much as we can, taking turns caring for them. It makes no financial sense to spend that kind of money if you can care for them at home.

This divide is very revealing about the economic history of this country and how it differs by race. When you work with this every day, sometimes you don't think about it. But sometimes, you stop for a minute and look around and you notice that these are all patients of Caucasian descent around you. You can see how this country works by looking at the different outcomes by race at the end of life. It's a window into the larger story of what life is like in the younger years as well and how it differs based on race. Many of the people of African descent are in government-paid facilities, not private ones.

As I travel around the world a lot and I see different treatment of seniors, I can make comparisons on the human condition that are broader than if I only looked at the United States.

One observation I have made is that staff members seem to give more respect and attention to residents whose family members are highly involved in their care, who visit often. I am including this in the book because I want you, the reader, to get a broader picture not just of nursing homes and assisted living, but of humanity, both the good and bad.

Maybe it can help bring some humanity back.

BALANCING
LOVE AND RESPECT

I'M NOT GOING TO SAY EVERY FACILITY IS BAD. I'M SURE there are some good ones out there. But speaking from my personal experience, the bad starts from the top because some owners are unscrupulous. They do not care about humans. All they care about is the dollar.

It's sad and sickening. Realistically, they know that when you push the caregivers—they're able to do the work. The owners and even some managers and CEOs don't know how to touch or answer a call bell. They walk around with authority but with no connection to the resident that is paying them thousands of dollars each month.

Some people pay fifteen thousand dollars per month for assisted living, and what they get in return from the owners is unbelievably little for that amount of money.

Caregivers in the United States are from countries all over the world. The way they treat patients usually is directly related to their cultural backgrounds back home. Caregivers from the islands, Africa, or even Europe bring something different to the table. Even with the low pay and stress of the job, they still bring morality to the job and respect for elders that sets them apart from others. This is not always an easy task under the stressful work conditions we have. But I have seen many caregivers hold up under the stress, supported by the moral ground they received in their home countries. That helps a lot.

HEARING GOOD STORIES

BUT I AM ALWAYS ENERGIZED BY THE HUMANITY OF THE residents who are very funny and nice people.

They come from all different walks of life. There are all different calibers of people. I've worked with people from homemakers to doctors, scientists, physicists, real Chicago gangsters, teachers, and PhDs.

These people all have different perspectives. It's a gift to be around them because you learn so much from them. They're interesting people who had interesting lives and the good thing is you hear good stories. You get to feel what they feel. The spark is still there. If they haven't given up, if they're angry, they're fighting back.

I have a resident who loves all the girls. He just goes crazy for girls. Every girl he sees, he'd say, "I love you, honey. You're beautiful." It's innocent. He'll tell ten women that he loves them. So stuff like that makes me laugh.

From their experiences, lifestyles, and from their environment, they bring new energy. When they touch you like that spiritually, you feel like you want to give back to them, no matter what the circumstances are.

Sometimes my coworkers get a little annoyed with me. I was working with this one lady and she used to be an ER nurse in New York. She likes sliced tomatoes, and some people didn't send it to the coordinator for the unit. They didn't put it in the system to let dietary know that this lady likes sliced tomatoes and it's such a big bureaucracy to get the woman some of it and it aggravates me. This woman is paying so much here and all she wants is sliced tomatoes. I went to the coordinator and said, "Oh, man, can we put it in the system, because it's just sliced tomatoes?" I could go to the kitchen, but they don't allow the staff to go and just take things. But I don't see the big deal in this woman getting some sliced tomatoes. She enjoys that and she doesn't eat a lot of other things.

For the first couple of days, I went and got it. I think they sent one and it went right back to the same old system. This woman is not getting that and she's paying so much money.

You look at these people as human beings. These are actual human beings, unique individuals, with lives and stories.

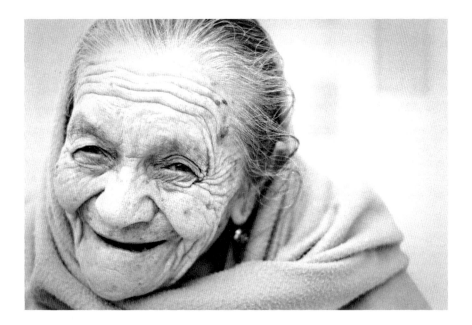

SELFLESS
FAMILY MEMBERS

I WILL GIVE SOME CREDIT TO THE FAMILY MEMBERS WHO are good.

There are family members that I've seen who really care. Every day, they are hands-on. They help their family members wash and shower and they will bring supplies. They are on top of things and they take turns. There are three sisters and one mother in one particular family that I work with. Every day, they check in on the father and they get involved. They're on top of things, and they buy supplies.

Another resident was a math teacher and a scholar. He is not a very old guy and is still ambulatory. But he has Alzheimer's and dementia, and his brain is gone. He is able to follow a few commands.

His sister and brother look after him.

The sister, Barbara, is literally there every day, sometimes twice a day. Maybe her lifestyle makes it easy and comfortable for her to do that. She lives close by.

Her brother's room is fully equipped with whatever he needs. The clothes are nice. She administers the drugs her brother needs, bringing them with her directly from the doctor. She has a camera on her phone in case she needs it. In short, she is doing all the right things.

She is very energetic. She takes him out for lunch. The staff members sometimes get annoyed by her because she is very comfortable hanging out at the facility. Tired staff members are going to find something to complain about when someone is active and all over the place. We see a lot of her. It gets on some people's nerves. But I think she gets on people's nerves for the right reasons. If she wants something for her brother, she will go and get it instead of waiting for the staff to bring it to her. She does what she has to do. I admire her for paying attention to everything that relates to her brother. She follows up on everything from laundry to medication.

For years and years, she has demanded that staff call her at 8 p.m. each night so that she can say goodnight to her brother. If you don't call her, she will call the facility and say, "I did not hear from him." One time, the call was dropped and she called and called back to find out what happened. I've never seen that with any other patient's family member. It's love like I have never seen. Her other brother also comes in and they take turns with the care duties. They are very well-off financially and can afford to do so.

In addition to caring for her brother, Barbara also volunteers to help with activities at the facility.

My hat is off to her. She may be annoying but she is annoying for the right reasons.

Many families can't put in that kind of effort. But it always helps if family members are pleasant, if they know how to talk to the staff; they don't feel like the world owes them everything and they're above people. When they're very nice and pleasant, it helps everybody. It helps their family members who are in our care.

RECOGNIZING MY WORK AND EFFORT

I HAVE BEEN REWARDED BY MY EMPLOYERS OVER THE years for making the extra effort and for caring for the patients. A couple of times I have been named employee of the month or given free trips for going beyond the call of duty.

I recently had a family member, a daughter, who called the corporate office to give me a compliment. I'm not perfect but I try to do what I can do. When I look at them, I see myself, I see my future or where I'm heading. I have to do what I can do.

However, one thing I have noticed during the COVID-19 pandemic is that facilities are so desperate for staff that they will pay new hires, right off the street, the same as someone who has been there ten to fifteen years. Say, you started at nine dollars an hour fifteen years ago and you are now up to fifteen dollars. Someone just starting is also paid fifteen dollars an hour. It's mind-boggling. But when you think about it from a business perspective, the owners of the facilities are not there to improve your life. The purpose is to make a profit. Whatever they have to do to make a profit, they will do that. They need stable staff. If that means paying a new hire the same as a veteran worker, they are going to do that. The demand for staffing is very high. If new staff demands seventeen dollars an hour, they are going to get it.

It's a vicious cycle that doesn't take humanity into account. But if you choose to work for someone else instead of having your own business, you can expect all of this. Everyone is disposable. It's not about humanity, it's about the budget. It's about managing the business in a way that will produce a profit for the owners.

In some facilities, if a resident oversleeps and misses breakfast and they request a tray to be delivered to their room, there is a nine-dollar charge to do that.

BEING CONSERVATIVE

IF ONE OF MY PATIENTS DIES, I USUALLY DON'T GO TO the funeral. There are some caregivers that do that but for me, coming from another culture and based on my mentality, I think it's the family's time for privacy. I think it's a time when the family needs to come together. It's okay if you're invited, but I'm from a culture where you do not push unless you're invited.

In my culture, in Jamaica, believe it or not, we're conservatives. We have a lot in common with Republicans and people may not realize that.

NURSING ASSISTANTS
AND WHO THEY ARE

I THINK IT'S IMPORTANT TO DISCUSS WHO NURSING assistants are.

They are caregivers. These are people, mostly from Third World countries, and I hate saying that because that's separating people. But that would be the word that people use to describe them. They're mostly from Africa, the Caribbean, and Spanish-speaking countries. You will not find someone from France or Germany.

You may find a few, one or two people, from the Czech Republic or Russia. These people come to America for different socio-economic reasons. They come for better opportunities, but they come with their strict morals and beliefs system from their home countries. They come with open-mindedness, they come with love and they come with mostly a lot of respect. In these countries, respect for the elders is the foundation of their existence. In Africa, speaking as an African-Jamaican person, you don't disrespect your elders. Even right now, when I'm walking past someone that is older, I hold my head up to acknowledge the person and I would say good morning or hello. That was ingrained in me when I was a child.

We come here from all these other countries with strong moral beliefs. A lot of caregivers have a religious upbringing. They are either Christians or Muslims, with very strong morals. When we come into a country where we see how our elders are living, it's a bit of a shock to us. Then the good inside of us kicks in. We have to show them respect and care based on our upbringing. It's kind of unusual to see it, but we get involved.

I've seen CNAs who have gone on to medical school. Some were police officers before coming to this country. They come to the U.S. for better opportunities because their country economically is not up to par. They don't have a bright future economically, so they come here. But these are smart people.

I've known CNAs who have huge houses back home. If they were living back there, they would be like kings and queens compared to people living in an apartment here. These people are very hardworking, very dedicated, and very strong people with good upbringing. But everyone wants to come to the United States based on what they hear about the economy and opportunities.

EFFECTS OF
WORKING OVERTIME

NURSING HOME STAFF MEMBERS, MYSELF INCLUDED, work very long hours. Even to this day, I work 188–190 hours over two weeks. That is normal for a lot of people in the industry. We want to achieve, earn, and take care of our family.

Some caregivers will work 188–190 hours at a nursing home then do a private duty as well. They may only go into a person's home, get them breakfast, run maybe some small errands, and then they leave.

We work six or even seven days a week. It is nonstop working.

But that has side effects, particularly on your health. Your body is running down. You definitely will get burned out. You end up frustrated. You gain weight because you're not able to cook good food. You end up eating food from the job. Mostly they give you food that has a lot of calories and fat.

Caregivers end up gaining a lot of weight. They overeat for so-called energy. They don't get to see their kids or raise their kids. Their kids grow up fast without seeing them because they are so caught up in working overtime just to meet their needs.

I have literally seen it destroy families. I have seen many extra-marital affairs happen because the caregiver was always at work. Then there is the stress of financial problems as well. Sometimes this spills over into the workplace with fights, accusations, divorces. There are kids who rarely see their parents because they are almost always at work. The parents bring the paycheck home but are rarely around. They are always working overtime. It literally defeats the purpose of trying to build a family and a life. One must be careful to manage their life and establish a balance so that work does not consume their life totally.

I am trying myself to cut back on my hours, to travel more and enjoy life.

These are the things that some caregivers have to go through. They're trying to maintain their lives and work a lot of hours to make a decent salary. They are making maybe $2,500, even $3,000, every two weeks. We can make money, but it comes at a price, physically and emotionally.

BACK INJURY

THE PHYSICAL EXERTION FROM THE JOB TRICKLES down into your back, knees, and hips. One of the things that I've noticed after being in the business for twenty years is that most people leave the profession walking with a limp or with knee problems that need surgeries. They also have serious back problems from lifting and pulling people. You're always on your feet.

I'm working right now with people who can't stand straight at the medicine cart. They have to be leaning against it. There are different types of shoes that provide more support, but that is not enough.

When you are on your feet constantly for fifteen or twenty years, the body is not designed for that. When you are tired, it's very hard to remember to use proper body mechanics to lift.

A lot of residents can't walk. They don't have steady gait, and so you need to lift or transfer them for daily activity, or to go to the bathroom and to get up for breakfast. They have machines in some cases, but it's a time-sensitive issue. You're being rushed. You have this long list of thirteen to fifteen residents. You have no time to go get a machine. It's probably easier if you pull a coworker to help you, to grab someone to come and help you transport. If the person that is going to help me to transport cannot lift, and we don't do it in rhythm, one of our backs will be hurt.

When your back is shut, you're out. I advise people to stick to the care plan. If you have the lift machine to assist you, use it, because you can't work if your back is out. I've seen people out of work for months with bad backs. They are constantly in pain.

It's the owners who create this kind of work environment. I think they know that it is literally or mostly impossible to use the lift machines all the time. The workers, as always, adapt, overcome, and do the best they can.

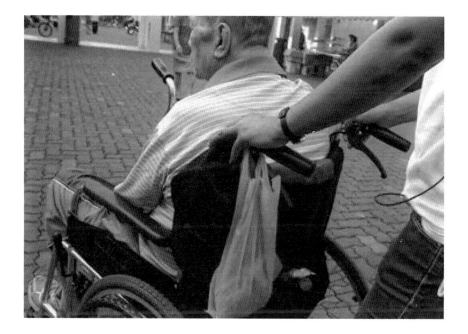

THE WEAR AND TEAR
OF BEING A CAREGIVER

LUCKILY, I DON'T HAVE ANY MAJOR BACK PROBLEMS yet. There's actually a little pain here and there on occasion. I try to be careful and do some exercises to strengthen my back. If you're not getting enough rest or sleep, that could be worse when it comes to dealing with residents.

I've seen the wear and tear of caregivers when they are stressed out. I've seen people develop mental health issues. I've noticed some of my coworkers' behavior and how they react to things, even with personal problems at home. It would trickle down. They developed behavior that is not consistent with rationality. They freak out about little things. They constantly yell about little things amongst each other, and not at the residents necessarily. They're burnt out and have no patience.

I've seen people having problems at home from overwork. They're not getting any sleep at all. Some would say, "Ian, my brain is not here right now."

They're totally tired and they say things that make no sense and they later come back and apologize for it.

Standing on your feet for hours every day on end takes a physical toll in addition to the strain of lifting patients in and out of their beds and wheelchairs.

I have seen many caregivers who eventually required back surgery. I have seen others who retire physically damaged because of the job. One has to be very careful.

The wear and tear of being a caregiver are vast. People who leave their family members in nursing homes don't realize the amount of stress the employees are going through. Some family members contribute to the stress. Some of them don't visit but maybe once or twice a year. And when they come, it is based on guilt, and they want to take it out on the caregiver. They stress you out and ask, "Why is my mother like this?"

They may not have seen the relative in a year. The residents may not have the necessary clothes that fit. There's no hygienic stuff that they bring and then they want to blame you for that. When you're short of staff, you would not even have time to shave somebody. Then, one day the family member comes and says, "Why is my dad not shaved?" So you have to keep your cool, or you will lose your job.

GUILT TRIP

IT'S A PART OF THE GUILT TRIP THAT THEY'RE ON. THE family doesn't want to be there. It's hard culturally, but, for me to understand because we don't have that in my country, I try to put myself in this position a little bit. The family doesn't want to be there. The resident doesn't want to be there. They feel guilty and they want to be superman or superwoman on that one day.

If you're there regularly, on top of the care of your family and you find something, you have more credibility in my eyes because you're there. I can see when you're involved. With that, I would say, "We apologize. We're gonna take care of it now."

You don't get aggravated because you know that this family member is always here. But the ones that show up once or twice a year, they have no credibility in our eyes. If they come in with an attitude, we just roll our eyes and think, "Get the hell out of here."

In our minds, we can talk back. They have no credibility with family members.

Overall, as far as the caregivers, from the start, it's just so much that we have to go through just for a paycheck.

BEING HUMAN AGAIN

IT'S GOOD TO START GOING BACK TO THINKING AND being human again, as it relates to when you're taking care of your mother, father, grandmother, or your grandfather, and see the situation that you're putting them in. Who will be dealing with them, and how will you treat them and act towards them? All of these, in a compilation, can be positive if you understand that, "This is my mother. She took care of me when I was a baby and she worked really hard."

What are we going to do now that she's not able to move? Those decisions have to be made consciously for the comfortability of the last days of your mother and father. I don't think humans are fair for someone to suffer in their last days if they took care of you as a baby. I don't want to be judgmental of people in this country or other countries that have nursing homes. I try to have an open mind because people have jobs. But, at the end of the day, whatever reality you want to create, you can create it by what you put in your mind and make it a reality. I'm not saying I could change everybody in this country or a country that has a nursing facility. We create our own reality. My reality in my country, we take care of our own, and I don't want to compare both.

Maybe the definition of love is money and finance for some people. It's doable, especially in rich countries. It's kind of hard for me to watch that also because I've seen where residents suffer on their last days—literally suffer in pain on their last days. It's something that I've seen regularly, and when I say suffer, that is because they're not home.

MULTITASKING

WHEN YOU'RE IN A PUBLIC PLACE OR FACILITY, PEOPLE need to keep in mind that you're dealing with many different residents with many needs. You don't have that one-on-one time to go sit with Miss Jane 24/7, to comfort her, or to see why she is in pain. There are so many different factors.

For example, she has dementia or Alzheimer's and she's a risk to herself. When she gets up, she will fall and maybe break or hit her head on something. That means particular care because they're maybe 5 percent alert where they could say and understand stuff, but they have dementia, and then they cannot walk properly. You have to try to keep them in one place. People are trying to do that with a list of job duties because they don't only do caregiving.

The owners of these facilities now get rid of departments where they are compiling. They're trying to get the most bank for their book. They would get rid of housekeeping and laundry and they would have the caregivers do the sweeping and washing of the plates. The same person has to do all of these.

In a big nursing home, they do have kitchen help, but in assisted living, the words sound good, but it's just living. You still end up with seven or eight people so they let you do the garbage, the mopping, and all that stuff.

SURVIVAL

THERE'S A GOOD PERCENTAGE OF PEOPLE WHO JUST become immune or they disconnect because they see that they should be doing more for the patients, but they can't. They just don't have time. It's not like deep down they don't care. I rarely see a caregiver that doesn't care. It's conditioning your mind. In my mind, it's called survival. To survive in it, you have to just do what you can do and move on.

I would say most people work in this field because they're human. We're from backgrounds where people have morals, respect, and love for people.

There are residents that don't want a black person taking care of them because they are from that time zone. There are men that have issues like violence. There are different situations mentally. They fight, they curse, and speak at you. On the other hand, they're funny, they're nice, and they're sweet. It's a variety of different personalities you have to deal with, from different times.

Sometimes they curse me out but it's so funny the way they talk. Sometimes, they think the building is their house and then say, "What are you people doing here? You're not paying any rent. Get out. This is my house."

We joke back with them respectfully and we laugh. That's the only mental break you have, a couple of minutes when someone is funny.

THINKING CAREFULLY

IN CHOOSING A NURSING FACILITY, FAMILY MEMBERS around the world need to think carefully about the human factor and the humanity in this choice.

When you come into a facility, be nice. It goes a long way when we have family members that are nice and considerate. In return, the caregivers will pass that consideration on to the family that we are caring for.

Please remember that while we are taking care of your relative, we often don't have time to see our own families.

I also think that people should consider keeping family members at home as much as they can, taking turns if necessary, before taking the step of putting them in a nursing home.

MONEY-DRIVEN DECISION

A LOT OF THE PEOPLE I TAKE CARE OF HAVE GOOD SAV-
ings. I don't see the rationality where people are spending so much money
on assisted living.

People don't understand that in assisted living, they take residents
based on the amount of money they have and how long they're going to last.
They do not accept you just because they have an opening and you're a nice
person. It's a money-driven decision when they take you into these homes.

I know people who are paying up to half a million dollars for assisted
living. When their money runs out, Medicaid kicks in. That's the agreement
initially.

But that doesn't happen. The heartbreaking part of it is, they get thrown
out or they have to leave when the money runs out.

The sad part is that you can spend half a million dollars over two years,
and still not get the care that you expect and deserve. The food is all pro-
cessed. There's nothing organic. There's no nutrition in it. It's just very fatty,
saturated bacon, sausage, powdered eggs, and toast. The only thing that has
some value is maybe some fresh vegetables and yogurt. Spending so much
to get so little makes no sense.

FINDING A SOLUTION

FAMILY MEMBERS SHOULD THINK BEFORE THEY BRING their family to a nursing home. They should have a game plan. The owners of these facilities need to stop thinking about money first.

In my twenty years of experience, I have found that owners do not care. They know that in order to provide proper care, you have to spend money to have proper staffing. But all they're thinking about is the profit. They're not thinking about actual residents that are suffering. I would conclude that they don't care.

At the end of the day, it's all about money. The only person who cares from the heart is the caregiver and some family members.

HEARTBREAKING SITUATION

A LOT OF THE FAMILY MEMBERS CAN'T DEAL WITH THIS.
It's easier for them to put them in a facility and spend the money. It's a very sad situation and I tried to see the good in it as best as I can. I just want people around the world to treat their family members better; be considerate. Think back to when you were a baby and the choices they made for you as a child. Try to make some of the same choices.

When they get older, they're vulnerable; they don't know who they are, and they're dealing with people that are burnt out, tired, and underpaid.

I just heard of one story the other day where nursing home workers had a thing called a "fight club." They make residents fight and they bet money. There are a lot of horror stories out there that I can't even get into. Luckily, I don't get to see a lot of these stories. Anything that I see that has to do with abuse, I report it immediately.

I see little things as far as family members or burned-out workers are concerned with direct abuse and always get it reported. The facility or the state nursing board takes care of that. In general, I just want people to be careful about how they are, how they treat their family members, and their decisions.

SOMETHING TO THINK ABOUT

JAMAICA IS NOT EVEN CLOSE WHEN IT COMES TO BEING rich, like America, but we do not have too many people suffering from dementia or Alzheimer's there. I see so many of those here. I'm so confused about why so many elderly people have dementia all the time in the U.S. but in Jamaica, I can't even think of one person who has it.

I have grandmothers and I know old people up to hundred years or more that still get up, make breakfast in the morning, and go out and do farming. They just get old gracefully. I'm sure there's a little bit of forgetfulness, but the severity of dementia and Alzheimer's in some persons versus Jamaica is not even close.

People need to research this. It may be a cultural issue.

MY PERSONAL
PHILOSOPHY ON AGING

IN WEALTHY, INDUSTRIALIZED COUNTRIES, PEOPLE ARE
living longer but are not part of the family support system. Instead of living
at home and helping with the family, they are in institutions.

This has almost no historical precedent. We are making up the rules
as we go. From where I sit, it looks like we are not doing a very good job.
Retirement homes are destructively expensive and can be socially isolating.
They are built for efficiency rather than quality of life. They are part of the
bureaucratic American health-care system and not an integrated component
of day-to-day life.

Philosophers don't really talk much about aging. Aging highlights the
frailty of the body.

We celebrate the virtue of youthfulness, glorifying the young and
able-bodied, giving preference to what others can do for us rather than
what we can do for them. We want excitement and activity, not calmness. We
want engagement in the moment. We want to be reminded of the potential
of youth, not the memory of things already done.

These are philosophical choices that need to be articulated and examined.

For society, aging is a practical, not a philosophical, endeavor. It's a
cumbersome and frightening process that needs to be managed. But like all
practical situations, it hides deep assumptions about its value and what we
take for granted. Our task is to reveal them, to ask how we can conceptualize
it all so that we can make the most ethical choices for ourselves and others.

Aging is inevitable, but our attitude towards it doesn't have to be.

A positive aspect of aging is that by the time we reach our senior years, we have a wealth of experience to guide us and we can confidently face whatever life brings our way. We become wiser about life, relationships, going through hard times, and so much more.

What is aging? It's a physical process that will always be with us. But the perception of aging and the views about the contributions of elders to society and what society owes them changes from era to era and differs from culture to culture.

Researchers at Johns Hopkins University came up with some interesting findings. They found the human aging process is special from a philosophical perspective in that only humans have the concept of aging. We know when we were born. We know that eventually we will die. We can look backward and forward in time and evaluate different stages in our lives. Other animals can't.

We wonder what this special human trait means for the pursuit of happiness and how to flourish in our lives. It opens up philosophical possibilities in our lives.

A philosophy of life is an overall attitude towards life and the purpose of human activity. Activities are limited by time and death. We forget this. We consume our time on distractions without asking if they are important or valuable.

That philosophy can evolve over time as a person sheds theoretical knowledge and gains practical knowledge; their personal vision and philosophy will also change.

WHEN RESIDENTS RUN OUT OF MONEY

I'VE SEEN PERSONALLY WHERE PEOPLE HAD TO LEAVE facilities because their money ran out. They were promised a Medicaid room after their money was all gone. When those two years pass, the nursing home says, "Oh, I'm sorry, we are done with you."

In assisted living, if you touch a resident's wheelchair and move it two feet, there's a charge for it. If you have to bring someone's food up, from the kitchen to the room, one-way costs nine dollars. That's just to bring the food up there. It is crazy.

If the resident chooses not to come down to the dining room, you take the food upstairs and that would cost nine dollars. You have to bring the floor trays for maybe six, seven, or eight people that don't want to come down today and they're charged for that.

Now they have tablets where the caregiver has to enter every single thing they do and you have options in the software to make more work. Everything there has a price. You as a caregiver don't see the price; you just enter a code.

For example, the resident is sitting in the dining room and they also have a TV room. From the TV room to the dining room, transporting them for ten steps has a price. Literally, once you touch them, you have to charge for it.

If someone is really not in the mood to go to bed that night, fights you, and is giving trouble in some ways, you would code it that way, and it's more money.

Your supervisor always asks, "Did you code for that? Did you put that in?"

They are so obsessed with coding.

The people from the corporate office come down and reiterate, "Listen, you guys have to code more. We need numbers."

The amount of work and staff you have is based on the amount of coding you do. If you're not coding, you're going to be short. That's greedy and sick.

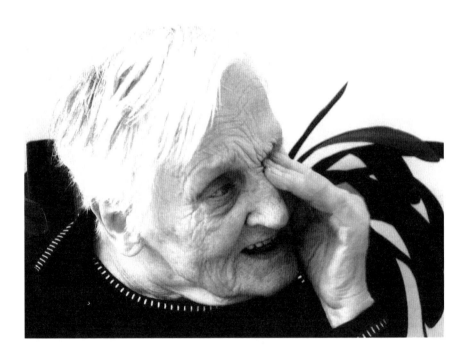

A GLOBAL PERSPECTIVE

AFTER TRAVELING AROUND THE WORLD TO DIFFERENT countries, I get to see what nursing homes are like from a cultural and a global perspective. I see how people treat their senior citizens or elderly differently from country to country.

In Africa for example, the elderly are revered and respected the older they get.

They look up to elders based on the fact that they worked hard and kept the family together. They value the wisdom that the elderly show us and teach us. They tell stories from when we were kids and pass on folklore. They teach us about legends or traditional medicine and how to be a man or a woman. They helped raise us physically and mentally.

They literally gave us life. In Ethiopia, if you want to marry someone, you have to go see your father, your spouse's father, and the village chief or leader of the village. These elders have the authority to approve the marriage or not.

In the United States, the elderly are not functional in society anymore. They are not given the power to make decisions as they are in other countries.

It's not just Africa, but basically a couple of countries that I've been to and have seen in Europe where the elderly are treated respectfully until their last days.

Another thing that I saw while in Africa was when an elderly person died, the entire town paraded and celebrated their life and death.

They come and mourn and go to the home of the person who passed away. On the day of the funeral, everybody comes out and they have a parade. Maybe we could learn something from this.

I would never generalize and say that all seniors are mistreated in the U.S. or anything because I've seen families here that are marvelous in the way they do things. I try my best to find positive things because, obviously, the United States is a different culture.

I try to be careful with my judgments. But I have to speak what I saw. I really feel strongly about how we treat the elderly in this country.

THE GOOD AND THE BAD

NURSING HOMES EMPLOY MILLIONS OF PEOPLE FROM around the world from all walks of life. If you live in the United States and you come from anywhere you can go to a nursing home and get a job. These are some of the good aspects of the industry. I've seen people that come here with nothing end up owning two houses, cars, and wealth from working at nursing homes. I don't have a big formal education, but I make over fifty thousand dollars a year. That includes a lot of overtime and hard work and being away from home. But it's still fifty thousand dollars a year, which is not a bad living.

A FLEXIBLE JOB

PEOPLE WORKING IN NURSING HOMES IN THE UNITED States send millions and millions of dollars back home to their families and relatives in their home countries. Nursing homes contribute a lot to the well-being of people around the world. You always have job security. I can take three or four months off to travel. As soon as I'm back, I get a phone call, "Hey, Ian, you're back in town; can you work Monday?"

You can keep multiple jobs if you're willing to work hard. It's a good business if you put some humanity into it.

I think, over the years, nursing homes are getting with the times as far as benefits such as health insurance are concerned. I've seen where caregivers are living better than doctors. If someone wants to go to school as a doctor, I've seen caregivers are living better than doctors.

FROM NOTHING
TO SOMETHING

IT IS AMAZING TO ME THAT SOME PEOPLE LOOK DOWN on a job like this. I travel the world. I have a nice car.

I get to learn Italian working in a nursing home. I didn't know anything about the Italian until I started working with older Italian residents. It's almost like one of the best jobs you can have because you get to interact with people. You're there with them on their last days of living. You get to see people on their journey from start to finish.

My experience as far as resident rights and abuse the law creates the guidelines for resident rights and abuse and all of that they created, but in reality, they create these rules and, well, which is it? I think the government guideline is good as to what to expect.

BEING HUMAN

THERE ARE GUIDELINES FOR RESIDENTS' RIGHTS AND abuse, but in reality, these rights are violated every single day. They are violated by the owners, by staff. Some of these violations are caused by staff burnout, lack of supplies, shortage of staff. It's a compilation of things. The rights are only as good as the owners make them.

We're talking about financial, sexual abuse. Any kind of abuse you could think of in the world goes on in nursing homes, period. It's a microcosm of the world. In a lot of cases, residents are abused from the first day they come into a nursing home until their last breath.

WHEN PRIVACY IS
TAKEN FOR GRANTED

ONE OF THEIR RIGHTS IS THE RIGHT TO PRIVACY. I HAVE SEEN
nursing homes where they do their best to protect privacy but others that don't.

You're supposed to knock the door when you go into a resident's room
but when you have thirteen, fourteen, or fifteen people in your care, you don't
have time to knock doors. I am not perfect either when it comes to pulling
curtains, knocking on a door, and stuff like that. Since I've been in this business for over twenty years, I never had—and I want my readers to understand
it, I've never had one problem with abuse. I have never been written up for
violating rights. I just thank God for that.

No matter how good you are, I've seen situations where you can't avoid
getting in some type of trouble. Residents are combative residents. You are tired.
You worked sixteen hours the previous day and are scheduled for another sixteen today. You're in a bad mood. You have situations at home that are stressing
you out. A resident throws water on you or calls you the "n" word.

This is a microcosm of the human condition. Anything can happen
in one of these places, but again, let's take into consideration the age, their
diagnosis, and all that. In work, you still respect them.

I've been able to survive all these years with not a single complaint,
because of my personality. I'm usually very calm in any situation. My grandmother says, "Put your mind to your condition." I walk around with that
mentality every day. When I leave my house and go to work, I try to remind
myself that you're going to take care of other people, with their different
personalities, and that no matter what comes, I need the job.

MENTAL AND PHYSICAL ABUSE BY RESIDENTS TO CAREGIVERS

PEOPLE SEE CAREGIVERS COMING TO WORK EVERY DAY with a smile. It's actually a requirement of the job, to smile at family members and residents, which is good because you need that smile to keep positive energy. But if they only knew the pain and suffering that we endure in our jobs. People don't realize the suffering and pain caregivers go through every day, all the while keeping a smile on our face.

In many cases, caregivers are overworked and are facing pressures at home as a result of being away so much and working on holidays and weekends. At work, they have to deal with physical and mental abuse from the people they are caring for, their family members, or their supervisor, their so-called "bosses."

We are told all the time that we are the "heroes," the front-line workers, the eyes and ears of the organization. But at the same time, we are underpaid and abused. There is serious hypocrisy going on here.

I've seen family members report us to our supervisors *because* we were nice to them. One was a daughter of a resident. She walked in and the staff was nice to her and polite, trying to get her up to speed on what she needed to know about her father. She complained to the administrator that were being *too* helpful, that were overdoing it. The administrator came back to talk to us, not admonishing us. It was civil but the fact that it came up in a staff meeting really surprised me. I had never seen that before, where you were trying to be nice to a patient or their relative and they didn't like it. There are some very strange people in the world out there that you have to deal with. You have to deal with emotions, with racist people. It's a lot. When you come home to your family and you finally get a chance to sit with your family at the dinner table and you relay what has happened at work, your family members question why you would ever want to go back there to face so much abuse. But the job puts food on the table and pays the bills. A lot of caregivers have no choice but to work there, basically. They typically don't have the education or skills to find another job that would pay as much. As I mentioned earlier, the pay is good if you are willing to work hard and long hours. But you have to be physically and mentally strong to do it. Sometimes you will have a shift that starts at 6 a.m. or 7 a.m. You have worked a double shift the day before, so you come to work already tired.

As I mentioned, almost everything is now the responsibility of the caregiver, even the laundry, as owners cut costs.

As you are working hard, managing all these tasks, exhausted, missing your family, you are sometimes subjected to racial slurs from the residents. They called you a nigger.

You have to remind yourself that these are the residents who still have the mindset from a different time. I try to have empathy for a resident who doesn't have the ability to even go to the bathroom by themselves or feed themselves. But yet, they still have the presence of mind to hurl a racial slur at you. It's hard not to take that personally. I'm not a doctor or a psychologist but I am still trying to understand where that comes from, the ability to verbally abuse a caregiver when they are so powerless to do anything else, even go to the bathroom of feed themselves.

Residents can also be physically abusive. They scratch you. They spit on you. They curse at you. They treat you overall in a very inhumane way. It's a common occurrence. This happens to caregivers all over the United States every single day. I've seen female caregivers getting kicked in the stomach, getting scratched, having their wrists and ankle sprained. This physical abuse is on top of back problems you experience from working on your feet all day.

That's one of the reasons I'm writing this book so people can see the good, the bad, the ugly of the nursing-home world. While there is a lot of good, there is a lot of bad also. I want people to see this. I would like the reader to try to imagine themselves in that position.

I once worked at an assisted living center in an old, converted hotel in Lakewood, N.J. There are a lot of poor people in that area, drug addicts, those who were HIV positive. It was a good business opportunity for the owner, a musician in his early fifties. The state would refer residents to this old hotel, which the owner had partially renovated. It still looked like an old hotel from the 1960s. The owner took residents that other facilities rejected, and somehow, he passed state inspection even though there were so many violations it was unbelievable.

I was taking care of a guy, a fairly young person, and all of a sudden, he turned around and started fighting me. This was some senile, old person. He was a young guy with mental problems. I have long dreads but luckily, I had my hair in a turban. He grabbed me, pulled my dreads out, and started fighting me. As a human being, my instinct was to retaliate aggressively. I had to quickly ask myself if I should fight him like a regular attacker or hold back because he was a patient maybe with more rights than me. Maybe I could go to prison for fighting back. It was a mess.

I had to defend myself at least partially. I grabbed him and threw him against the wall. The owners of these facilities are often only concerned about making money, not about the danger they are creating for the caregivers. The mental and physical abuse of caregivers is widespread. Because we need to take care of our families, we suck it up and endure it. There are also, of course, many nice residents who are sweet and kind. But the problem is that many people with mental problems don't behave in a civilized manner. They aren't civilized beings.

Residents often look at caregivers as servants, "the help." When I do get a chance to have conversations with them, to tell them that I travel around the world and have lived around the world, including Ethiopia, Italy, and England, I have a child in France, they are shocked. Their eyes are opened wide.

"When did you become so intelligent?" one resident asked me.

When they use snarky, racist words for me, they do it almost as if they are joking. But I pity them. Sometimes I just let it go. It's not an easy thing to endure, mentally. But it's something you have to deal with every day as a caregiver.

Sometimes you will knowingly be sent into a room to help a resident who doesn't like "colored people." The resident won't tell you to get out, but they make your life a living hell. They look uncomfortable and angry no matter what you do to help them. And they will report you in a second to the supervisors because they don't like Black people. They scrutinize everything you do. They don't want you to be in the room too long because they think you are going to steal something. For the caregiver, it's mental torture.

In this field, if you get accused of anything by a resident, it's a big problem, even though the accusation later turns out to be false. It still has to be investigated.

The inconvenience that causes a caregiver is not a bed of roses. The building on the outside may look happy but the caregivers suffer with mental and physical abuse from everyone. I hate to sound like it's all bad. But it is a reality for the workers. I hope you, the reader, will understand the environment that your family members may be living in. I give credit to a lot of the residents for their strength in coping with all of what goes on every day in these facilities. There is a lot of suffering. It's horrible and inhumane in a lot of cases, based on my experiences.

DYING ALONE

OFTEN, I SEE RESIDENTS DYING ALONE WITH NO FAMILY members around them on their last days. The last person that they get to see is a caregiver. It makes me think a lot about humanity and the human condition.

These people spent their lives taking care of their families. And there's nobody there with them on their last days. It's horrible. I see myself in these residents as I watch them taking their last breaths. It's unbelievable.

There was one woman who tested negative for COVID-19 but there were other patients who tested positive; the daughter did not want to be exposed, so she let her mother die alone.

Her mother was dying and she decided to let her go. I was caring for that lady. It took her weeks to die.

She was there struggling. Sometimes when I went in to care for her, I had to give her a cotton swab with water because her mouth was dry.

You just don't let someone die like that. The daughter couldn't visit, but the staff, thinking that she had COVID-19 stayed away from her as well. Only assigned people could go in and care for her. I watched this lady just pass away.

I thought about her when she was younger, coming up in school, raising her family. Is this what life about?

I looked at her and I said goodbye in my mind because I knew tomorrow, she wouldn't be here.

I realized that life is unpredictable. It's very different. It's strange. It has its good and bad points. But the way our residents are being treated in a lot of cases is not fair and not right.

And it's not human, you know, and I just think people should pay more attention today.

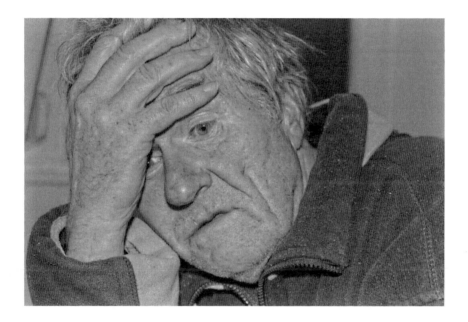

SOLUTIONS

AS WE WORK TO IMPROVE NURSING HOMES AND assisted living facilities, I think one of the first things one has to look at is their mentality towards the elderly, how you think the end of their lives should be, and what you can contribute to them, based on what they have given to you. This boils down to the humanity inside of you, your culture, and your views on what is unacceptable and what is unacceptable.

Often, it boils down to money. Family members don't have time for their elderly relatives because they are too busy making money. I don't see anything wrong with making money, but you are caught in a culture where everything is money driven, there are some side effects and casualties. Sometimes, the elderly are the casualties. They are neglected. In some cases, they are treated worse than animals. These are people who gave their all to raise their children and now they are being abused physically, emotionally, and financially.

Other cultures with much less money than ours seem to be able to take care of their elderly better than we do. It can be done. It comes down to personal choice. If less affluent societies can manage to accomplish better care with fewer resources then the wealthier societies can also do so, if we make that choice. First, you must make it a priority. In the United States, it does not seem to be as much of a priority as it is in other cultures. In the U.S., everyone in the family feels compelled to go out and work and make money. Nobody has the time for grandmother or grandfather. I have seen this in my personal experience. Relatives have gone years without visiting their loved ones. That tells me that their humanity is gone.

It depends on the culture. It depends on one's definition of love and how you want to give back.

In my work, I have seen good family members as well. They find the time and provide the care and attention their relatives deserve. That has given me hope that a solution is possible.

If you find yourself in a situation where you feel like you have no choice but to put your loved one in a facility, you and your family members have to *be there* as much as you can.

First, you must decide to get involved. Once you take them out of their house and into a facility, you are making a decision on how they will live for the rest of their lives. Will they spend their last years with respect, dignity, and peace? You and your other family members have to make the decision to be there physically, not just financially. That is the only way your relatives will be treated with the dignity they deserve in an assisted living facility.

Even then, it's not foolproof because you can't be at the facility all the time. You have to leave at the end of the day. You have placed your relative in a business. A business will never treat your family member as you do. Businesses are about money, not love.

I would suggest that before you place a loved one in a nursing home or assisted living center, have a family meeting and make a plan for how you are going to make this as comfortable as possible for your relative. Put some thought into the plan.

I know that this is not always easy, particularly if some family members live in different parts of the country. But it's also human. These are family members who devoted their entire lives for you to have a life. So when you make a plan, consider giving back as much you can to make sure they are as comfortable as they can be. To me, that is real love.

People can always find convenient excuses as to why they can't help out. They can easily lose sight of who this person was and what they sacrificed and contributed.

Make sure that everyone can contribute to Mom or Dad's transition. Let everyone take turns visiting them, maybe every other day. Work out a schedule, a program based on love, humanity, and what you are going to give back to your mother, father, or grandparents collectively.

Most people don't have a clue as to what actually goes on inside the facilities, what the residents eat, what they wear, what they see, how they feel.

After your loved one has been admitted to a facility, watch everything. Ask questions. Do your research. Read the reviews. Walk around the facility. Check things out. It's a process and it will take time.

Try to choose a facility that is convenient to everyone or at least as convenient as it can be. Once you pick the facility and you have done the background research, you will have to decide how to pay. There is Medicaid, Medicare, and private pay. And it can make a big difference.

If it's private pay, you can demand a lot more from the facility. You can have a say in everything. As I mentioned earlier, the minimum you are going to spend for private pay is probably around thirteen thousand dollars a month. For that, you deserve the very best and you can demand it. You have bargaining power. You have more choices for care, medication, security— basically everything.

But you must be specific about exactly what you want. And you still have to be personally involved. Just throwing money at it is not enough. Without personal involvement, you will be in the same situation as someone with no money.

The first thing I would advise is to go over with the facility about the legal rights of the residents. These are documents such as power of attorney, do not resuscitate, etc. Understand your rights and your family member's rights. You are entitled to get copies of any documents for your own records, including the resident's medical charts. Pay attention to any new medications or any other changes in their health care. There are people in facilities that systematically make choices on medication. It is often an automatic decision that is not necessarily based on the patient's best health needs. The facility should not make any health decisions without first consulting the family and without receiving their permission.

Take a day off work and go into the facility. Ask to see your relative's charts. Go through the care plan with a fine-toothed comb. Ask questions. Look around the resident's room. Watch the mannerisms of workers, how they approach you, how they speak. Check the timing of meals and the temperature of food when it is delivered.

Make full use of technology. If your relative is capable, they can have a cell phone with a camera to record abuse.

Just because you are paying top dollar for your relative's care does not mean they will be immune from abuse. I have seen many private-pay patients endure a lot of things that aren't very comfortable because of the lack of checks and balances and accountability. The ill treatment, even if it is not intentional, happens. I see it every day.

Remember, the owners are not in business because they are compassionate. They are in business to make money. There may be some humanity from the caregiver every once in a while. But when the caregiver is overworked, tired, and not given the resources they need to do the best job, humanity takes a back seat. That's just a reality.

It's about money and it's about timing. For the owners, the two are connected. Time is money.

If breakfast is supposed to be over at 9 a.m. and they start at 8 a.m., some residents will get skipped. They just don't eat. It's good to keep track of your relative's appetite and to ask them if what they are eating, particularly if they may be taking medication on an empty stomach. The goes for hydration. Make sure they are getting plenty of fluids. Make sure they are checked for urinary tract infections. Check for falls, and whether they are able to walk properly. I have seen that once a person falls and breaks a hip, they are never really the same.

I once cared for a patient, Nick, a retired school administrator. His was broken and his family didn't realize it. Every time they touched him, he was in a lot of pain. He was in excruciating pain for nearly three years before they finally realized it. The good thing was that his entire family was involved in his care and they were able to notice this and to eventually get him help. But they are not there every day.

A resident may appear nice, clean, with their hair combed when you visit. But there may be a lot of suffering going on that won't surface until after you leave. But it still helps to be there as much as possible. By the way, the staff are trained by management, not to talk too much about the resident's medical condition. They are supposed to refer you to supervisors. If you find a staff member who is honest with you, cherish that.

My advice: Be on top of everything. Show up. Monitor. You can do this in a nice, professional way. In particular, be nice to the staff. Don't have an attitude. But check everything. Make sure you are there on holidays and birthdays. The elderly often know when it is a holiday and they want to relive some of that. Don't just send a card. Be there with love.

Another area you need to monitor is recreation and socialization. This is important as you get old; all your friends and many of your relatives have died.

Give them food that reminds them of when they were at home cooking. Bring them their favorite foods. Consider taking them home for a weekend. Take them to church on Sunday. It can help them regain their dignity. You are restoring something from their earlier life that was peeled away as they grew old. Just driving to church and seeing the old neighborhoods can help. Seeing old friends at church can help as well. You would be surprised what a difference that makes emotionally.

Try to give them as much of a normal life as possible before they transition. If your intention is to help them live longer, this will definitely help because they feel like they are loved.

The hard work you put in will pay off.

This is a job that is too big for one family member alone. It's not a full-time job but it can take a lot of time. One person can't take on all the responsibility.

Set up a system among family members with dates and times, shifts. It's not easy. It takes time. Everyone is busy with their own lives. But giving back to your loved ones is only fair because they are the ones that gave you that life. They gave you everything.

This generation may feel like they don't owe anything to their relatives. A relative once told me, "I didn't sign up for this."

But the parents did not sign up for this initially either.

Once you have set up a system for supporting a loved one in a nursing home or assisted living center, and you and your relatives are hands-on and are involved, showing up every other day or as often as possible and pay attention to details, your loved one should be fine.

MY NAME IS FRANCIS: I HAVE DEMENTIA AND I'M LOST.

I SPENT HALF MY CAREER YEARS WORKING WITH Alzheimer's, dementia reminiscent, and memory-care patients. Sometimes, I wonder what goes through their minds. What is the thought process of a person with dementia or Alzheimer's? How do they feel? What are they thinking?

A lot of times I've seen them wandering. Were they looking for something or someone or trying to get out of the facility? Were they trying to find a family member, a job, or their car?

One patient, Francis, can verbalize her needs and wants. At times, she can hold a conversation intelligently. The next minute, everything that comes out of her mouth doesn't make any sense. That is a normal functionality of a brain with Alzheimer's.

I once asked to Francis, "How are you today?"

She stared directly in my eyes, looking at my facial expression. And in a low tone, she said, "I'm OK."

Her lips were kind of dry, so I told her I was going to get her something to drink, some cranberry juice. She said, "OK."

Now she was more comfortable with me having a conversation with her. She suddenly turned face-to-face with me and said, "Can you give me a ride home? I am looking for my baby. I am looking for my husband. I don't have my car with me; can you please help me?"

So I told her, "Francis, I will do whatever I can to make you feel comfortable and also to be honest with you."

Then I said to her, "Francis, how can I help you?"

She replied, "Am I dead? Is this real or a nightmare?"

And for a moment there, I started to get an insight into her thoughts.

She went on to say, "I don't feel anything. I don't know what to feel. I feel lost."

I looked her in the eyes and said, "Francis I'm going to be very honest with you just to try and help you gain an understanding of what's going on. Miss Francis, your husband passed away. You do not have a car. Your kids are all living in California at the moment and before they left, they put you in a nursing facility for you to be taken care of because your children have their own families, and they are not able to do it for you. You will be monitored and taken care of 24/7 around-the-clock with doctors and care managers to make sure that you're comfortable and safe. So that's why you are here in a nursing facility."

Francis then turned to look at me with both hands at her jaw, shocked and terrified that she lost her husband, her kids were not here, and she did not have a car or a job anymore.

She turned to me and said, "Oh my God, when did this happen?"

I said to her, "You've been here now going on two years and the facility has been doing a good job taking care of you. Your family loves you. They call you. If you recall, your daughter from California came by a few times to see you with your grandkids. So your family is still in touch but they have to take care of their own families and so they come to see you on holidays and on your birthday. Your family still loves you and thinks about you."

Then she said, "Oh my God, I can't believe this is happening. This is a *real* nightmare. My husband and I worked very hard to take care of our kids and family and all of a sudden, I'm in a place where people are telling me when to eat, when to shower, what to do, with no family members around me. I am feeling scared, alone, and abandoned. What is happening? Where is my family? I cannot leave. I feel like I'm placed under arrest. I don't feel free to go where I want to go. I can't believe this is happening to me. Oh my God."

So, I held her hands and said, "As your friend, I say everything is fine. You are OK. You are in good hands, OK? Your children make sure you're in a safe place where you will be taken care of. So, you have nothing to worry about."

Then she started to cry and said, "Please could you take me home? Could you take me home please? I need to go to my home."

I said, "Francis, there's no way I can take you out of this building because your family brought you here. I work here and I cannot take you home."

Understandably, Francis was irate and upset. She got up and walked away, calling for her husband and looking for her car and just wandering around searching.

I started to think deeper about the brain and some stories that were told by my grandmother and other people about spirits that wander. For some reason, in my mind, I was thinking along those lines and wondering if people with dementia Alzheimer's are lost souls wandering around searching for their loved ones.

They talk to people but the people do not understand. Just the thought of someone wandering around, searching but not being able to speak or understand is horrifying to me. In their minds, they know they had a family. They did not forget that. Just searching and looking for them without any explanation. Searching. Searching.

They know what they want to say but it's not coming out the right way and they're looking directly in your eyes and your facial expression but can't hold a conversation. And so, it becomes very frustrating for them and for the person that they're trying to talk to.

It is also very frustrating for them when they are trying to talk to someone and the person walks past them without acknowledging or answering them.

So, all one has to do is to put themselves in that situation and see how horrible it feels.

I tell the story of Francis simply because I want people to understand what the elderly with dementia Alzheimer's have to go through in their lives when they reach this stage in a nursing facility with no family, no friends. Everyone around them has died. They end up alone in a building with strangers.

I think if people put themselves in that scenario, they will probably treat the elderly a little better with more humanity.

FALLS:
THE LAND OF NO RETURN

TAKE MY HUMBLE ADVICE. IF YOU HAVE A LOVED ONE
living in a nursing home or an assisted living facility, please do everything
in your power to not let them fall.

I do understand that falls are unavoidable in many cases and beyond
your control. Facilities tend to have floors with hard surfaces such as tile,
which are easier to clean and are smooth for easier mobility. But they are also
more damaging for falls than, say, rubber mats or carpet would be.

But the reason I'm writing about this is just the pain and suffering physically and psychologically they have to go through when they fall. From my
experience, most residents never come back the same to the way they were
before they fell.

And this, in my opinion, is because of multiple medications they are
taking, their frail systems, lack of movement, and a variety of natural reasons. I do understand that there are laws that prohibit the unnecessary use
of restraints unless there is an emergency situation. Residents have the right
to be free from any form of restraint.

Restraints can also cause physical damage such as loss of bone, muscle
mass, mental depression, and constipation.

I've also seen chemical restraints that have been used. Residents who are
given these look sleepy, lethargic, and out of it. They also refuse meals because
they're always sleeping or have no appetite. And that, in itself, causes a whole
list of medical issues because you're not eating and not properly hydrated.

So, in most cases, restraints don't really work. No matter what direction you go as it relates to protecting your loved one from falling, the resident is going to have serious problems unless you're on top of things and have twenty-four-hour monitoring.

And there are many ways you can monitor your relative, such as taking turns with family members visiting. Or, you can do electronic monitoring from home, work, or anywhere.

I know for a fact that most nurses find it easier to give a resident who complains of pain a Tylenol or pain medication, despite the side effects. And because of the resident's age and medical condition, it doesn't really relieve the pain.

It's also important to choose a facility that is fully staffed. Even though a facility may have a policy against using restraints, there will still be broken bones and fractured hips if there isn't enough staff on hand to make sure residents don't fall.

I also suggest working with the physical therapy department on ways to help prevent falls.

I understand most families don't have the resources and funding to have round-the-clock care to help avoid accidents.

But what puzzles me is that I see a lot of family members who *do* have more than enough financial resources to afford good care around-the-clock but *still* put their family members in a facility.

When a resident does fall, the sudden shock and trauma create problems both physically and psychologically that change their attitude and mood.

As a caregiver, it's very hard for me to watch because everything changes for them, and they usually begin deteriorating. It really is a slide into the land of no return.

"I OUTLIVED MY SAVINGS: SOME WANT ME TO HURRY UP AND DIE"

I NEVER THOUGHT I WOULD LIVE TO SEE OR HEAR FAM-ily members, loved ones, organizations, and staff members say that they that would want a resident in a nursing home or assisted living to "hurry up and die."

During my career of up to twenty years as a caregiver, I've seen it and heard it but I have not wrapped my head around that thought, idea, or mentality because I'm from a culture where that is almost impossible. So it's kind of a shock to my brain.

It is only recently that I thought of digging in deeper in order to understand what this phenomenon is. After multiple interviews and research, I came to realize it is a complex situation and that I have to be careful in judging people. In the American culture, there are many sides to a story. That is the reason why I say it is complex because we are living in a culture where there are many situational circumstances with different families and their social economics.

If I can see life from a cultural and a global perspective, it helps me to explain the American reality, as it relates to the elderly with a well-rounded perspective free of judgment.

I have to also have an open mind in trying to understand why people come to these decisions. I wanted to understand their mentality and their morality. Let's start with the family members that have good and loving intentions.

What I found in the testimonials I've received in my research and interviews is that it is hard for some family members to watch their elderly mother, father, or family members who cannot walk, talk, or who may have some type of disease or cancer that is terminal.

In many cases, they are suffering physically and mentally. And it is very hard for them to deal with that situation emotionally every day and watch their family members suffer. So, you will find family members who just don't want to see their elderly mother or father in such a bad state.

This is especially true if when they were younger, they used to have conversations with their children, telling them, "Don't let me suffer or go out in pain."

They were mentally able at that time to express those needs and desires. The children or relative would make promises that they would never let them suffer or go out in pain. And when that promise can't be kept, the relative suffers from guilt and it's just all around a very sad situation.

A combination of guilt, stress, personal circumstances, and financial hardship makes it more difficult. Sometimes it's too much to handle and families end up making decisions in their own interests. That doesn't mean they had that intent; it's just the way events evolved. And so from that standpoint, I didn't see or suspect any ulterior motive or special interest in their decision. It is just natural love and choices and the cards that they've been dealt. They are trying to do what is in the best of their loved ones.

Whenever the situation is approached with true, genuine love, I saw where the family members look helpless, sad, and just emotionally drained. Whenever they come to visit their loved ones, you could just see it in their eyes and body language. It's just a lot to deal with. As someone who observes and documents, I try to write with an open mind and understand without passing any judgment.

On the other hand, organizations with special interests and family members with ulterior motives make me sick to my stomach, to be honest. Let's start with the family members who are just heartless. I get to see them with my own eyes when they enter the facility.

The staff does not know how to approach or even show them a warm welcome because we haven't seen them come to visit in a long time. When their relative passes, they walk in with some type of guilt or mixed emotions, so it turns out to be a very tense, uncomfortable moment because we haven't seen them in a long time. If they start to ask questions about material stuff from estates and anything to do with money, that's a big turn-off.

For months and years, they never call or bring any form of hygienic supplies, soap, powder, or whatever someone would need. Even on holidays and birthdays, maybe they will send a birthday card once in a while and that's it. It's pathetic how these people could just put their family in a nursing facility and just disappear, only popping up towards the end of life.

Then they show up with a lot of guilt and act aggressively towards the staff. Then it becomes clear that what they really are interested in is the money or estate of the relative.

They start to do a big calculation and investigation about how much money is left in the bank account or in stocks or bonds. Then, they go into overdrive when they realize they may not end up not getting anything because there is nothing left.

If the relative is still alive, they will sometimes start making drastic decisions for the resident because all the money is being sucked up by the nursing home. They're not happy that the relative is alive and kicking, particularly if they bounce back from an apparent near-death situation.

I could understand this if the financial burden is overbearing and if the resident does not have any savings or assets to deal with their final bills and it's draining the pockets of their children and they are truly suffering. But from my experience, 99 percent of the residents in assisted living have some savings are money put away because most assisted living facilities will not accept them if they don't have assets or savings that exceed at least a half million dollars. So, these residents *do* have some money put away for their final days, plus life insurance and other insurance and hidden assets that the family knows about. All the family members are thinking about is what the resident is leaving to them and they show up just to claim all of that. It makes me sick cause then it sends a message that human beings are disposable. You just use them, throw them away, and take what they have.

Now, let's talk about cooperation facilities and management.

I was in my nursing office with a few staff members the other day. There were three staff members and a director of admissions, and they were talking about their experiences with family members, next of kin, and power of attorney. They were talking about how family members act when they see funds are being depleted and estates may be taken. They noted the frustration on the relatives' faces and how they ask, "Why isn't this over yet? Why is she still hanging on?"

They don't verbalize it, but the mannerisms and choice of words are self-explanatory. Sometimes they even act as if it's a joke. But you know it's coming from a place that is not very good.

As a caregiver that has engaged with hundreds or thousands of family members for so many years, after a while, you can tell when someone has ulterior motives, and personal agendas.

And if their behavior is coming from a place of greed. Sometimes the humanity in me wants to just say, "Stop. What you're doing is not right." But I hold my tongue. Otherwise, I could lose my job.

I am not saying this does not happen in any other cultures, but I have traveled around the world and have never seen it in any parts of Europe, Africa, and especially my country, Jamaica. So I don't know if it's a cultural system in the United States or if it's a human condition or just simply a mental issue.

I have seen a lot of cases where a family member was preparing for the resident to pass. They have Catholic priests. They have everything ready. The chemistry of the residents' rooms was dark and sad; the staff and everyone were bracing and prepared for the resident to expire. Then, in a day or two, the resident would just get up, walk around, and order what they want to eat, totally back to normal. So we cannot predict mother nature. Now let's talk about management and some staff.

This part for me is one of the hardest parts to digest. Once I was in my supervisor's office and she and the wing nurse were having a conversation about a resident who kept bouncing back from being close to death. She was physically active, walking, talking, so the supervisor was frustrated. She is a professional and she knows what she's doing, but for me, it is very hard to wrap my head around it because I know her to be a very nice, seemingly caring person.

She was acting within the law, but she also has room for discretion.

The family and doctors decided to turn off the heart defibrillator machine the resident was wearing inside her chest. They also gave orders to stop pushing certain types of fluids and nutrients, but this lady was still walking around actively, trying to communicate, and walking even looking better, stronger than the rest of the residents in this facility. She was not going anywhere and so in the conversation, the supervisor was telling the wing nurse, "Maybe we should up the morphine with Ativan because both morphine and Ativan would slow her system down."

She would not feel any pain based on what the charge nurse said. I think she was acting under the authority of family members.

The fact that this was even being suggested while I was standing there was shocking to me. I could not process it because through the window, I could see that poor woman still walking around, looking exhausted and out of breath.

Even with her heart machine turned off but she's still moving around very strongly and trying to communicate. That blew my mind. I know with 100 percent surety that the supervisor and the family members don't have evil intent or malice or anything towards the resident. They were just following the protocol from the doctors. But in the back of my mind, I still think they have room for discretion or some type of mercy. My supervisor jokingly looked at her watch and said, "Hurry up already," with a laugh. I don't think she realized what she did because it was so automatic and to be honest with you, she was very stressed out with the amount of workload that they put on her. It's just one of those routine procedures.

These decisions and processes seem very complicated. I'm just a caregiver and I don't know the legal processes or even the rights of family members and all the rights that a resident has when it comes to the end of life. But in lay terms, I still can't process that entire situation.

I just want to get this off my chest and beg people in this society around the world and for those reading this book to please show your elderly relatives more love, care, and respect.

It is not nice to treat the elderly in this fashion, to deprive them of any comfort at the end of their lives, to turn off machines that would extend their lives, to stop giving fluids, to cut off all life support because you are frustrated, or you can't deal with it. It is not human.

I'm asking people to prioritize plans for their elderly when they reach the end of life. It's simply not fair to treat them this way. They did not do that to you when you were a baby and when you were sick. They sacrificed their entire lives for you. In some cases, they missed out on college or careers to take care of you and now you're in a rush to end your life because of financial gain.

To the families that truly have no choice and have their backs against the wall financially and do not want to see the suffering of their loved ones, I support you and I respect you.

For some of my staff and coworkers, it is not your place to make judgment calls on someone's end of life based on your own feelings or opinions. You wouldn't like that to be done to you. You are there to show compassion, give care and make a resident comfortable.

I hope at some point in this country and culture we would start to prioritize love over profit.

CONCLUSION: ARE YOU PREPARED FOR YOUR END OF JOURNEY IN A NURSING FACILITY?

I ASK MYSELF THIS QUESTION A LOT AS I AGE. I THINK about it a lot.

Did I save enough money? Do I have any assets? Do I have an estate? What will my financial security be when I become an elder if my loved one chooses to put me in a nursing home or assisted living? What would the rest of my life be like?

When I think about these questions, I feel terrified, scared, and helpless, especially knowing what I know now as the author of this book based on dozens of interviews testimonials, research, and experiences.

We, as baby boomers and younger people, are walking around enjoying life right now which is a good thing. Some of us are now enjoying life without a care in the world, not thinking about the end of the road.

But when you reach a certain age—seventy, seventy-five, eighty, or ninety—the reality will kick in. It will be even worse if your children or next of kin are not in any position to take care of you when you become incontinent, when you're not able to walk, when you're not able to speak, when you're not independent anymore.

They have their own lives and responsibilities and then they are faced with an entirely new set of obligations when they have to put you in a nursing home.

But before we get to that part, first you have to think about what kind of savings you have to live comfortably in a nursing home if your family is not able to keep you at home. And I say this within the context of the culture we are living in in the United States, where most people's minds are conditioned around earning money and wanting to become successful. With that success comes responsibility and you may not have time for what truly matters.

Most people's lives are taken up with their own affairs, responsibilities, problems, and with them trying to figure out solutions. So, the thought of taking care of you and having the resources to take care of you when you get older doesn't really cross their minds.

They are overwhelmed by the stress of paying bills and other issues. Their time is devoted to surviving in this culture.

Do you have fourteen thousand dollars or more per month to take care of yourself in an assisted living center or nursing home?

I have never worked in a state-run facility but from what I hear, there are many problems there. Are you prepared mentally for what is coming? In this culture, this is exactly what is going to happen unless you're lucky to have a good family that keeps you home.

Currently, 4.5 percent of elder adults—about 1.5 million—live in a nursing home and around one million in assisted living. About one out of three adults over the age of sixty-five are living in a nursing home at least temporarily.

There is a 40 percent chance of you or your loved one spending some time in a nursing facility. So, plan ahead. Use critical thinking to look into different options. Pay very close attention to every single detail.

If you know that this will be your destination when you reach a certain age, it is important that you start planning with your now. Otherwise, you will be shocked, hurt, and disappointed if this is not properly planned with your children or other family members.

We never think of these things when we're in our youth, healthy, and strong and young. But those inevitabilities always sneak up on you. If you are not prepared then you have a problem.

Ending up in a nursing home is probably the furthest thing from your mind. You probably can't imagine being in a nursing facility with no friends, no family, and in some cases no contact with the outside world. All your friends and family have died. You start to feel isolated, scared, powerless, and you lose your independence. All of that is overwhelming on the mind.

Some residents whom I interviewed for this book said they really didn't plan on living in a nursing home. It just happened suddenly. And in a lot of cases, they did not have any say in the matter. Any planning was almost overnight. It just happened suddenly. But at least they had financial backing, money that they saved, assets, and in some cases, good families. That helped make the transition a little smoother.

Take my humble advice and start to prepare for this part in your journey.

Prepare yourself for a complete change in your lifestyle, your surroundings, and in everything else. When you get older, you're not able to express your feelings, not able to walk or talk.

With no family members around, you are in a very dangerous situation. I can tell you right now, it's a totally different world from where you're living right now, when you are healthy and strong.

I am not trying to scare anyone. I'm simply telling you my experience working in this environment for more than twenty years and what I've seen. So, if I can help someone to be prepared as they approach the end of their journey then I would have done my part in educating people about the inner workings of a nursing facility so they can make better decisions when they reach that age.

Let me be clear and a little bit more open about my personal situation.

I don't have any plans myself for growing old. I think about it every day. As of now, I do not have the financial resource and I don't know what is going to happen.

My situation is not dissimilar from many other people. So, it is a scary thought and a scary reality.

I must, however, try to at least make sure I have good, compassionate people around me such as my children and a good wife. I am still young, strong, and healthy, so at least I may have some type of security, the kind that comes from love around me.

So, take my humble advice and prepare yourself for your end days in a nursing facility.

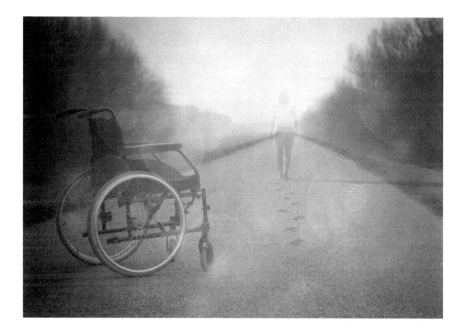